Heaven's Edge

A Story of Hope in the Darkness of OCD, Anxiety & Depression

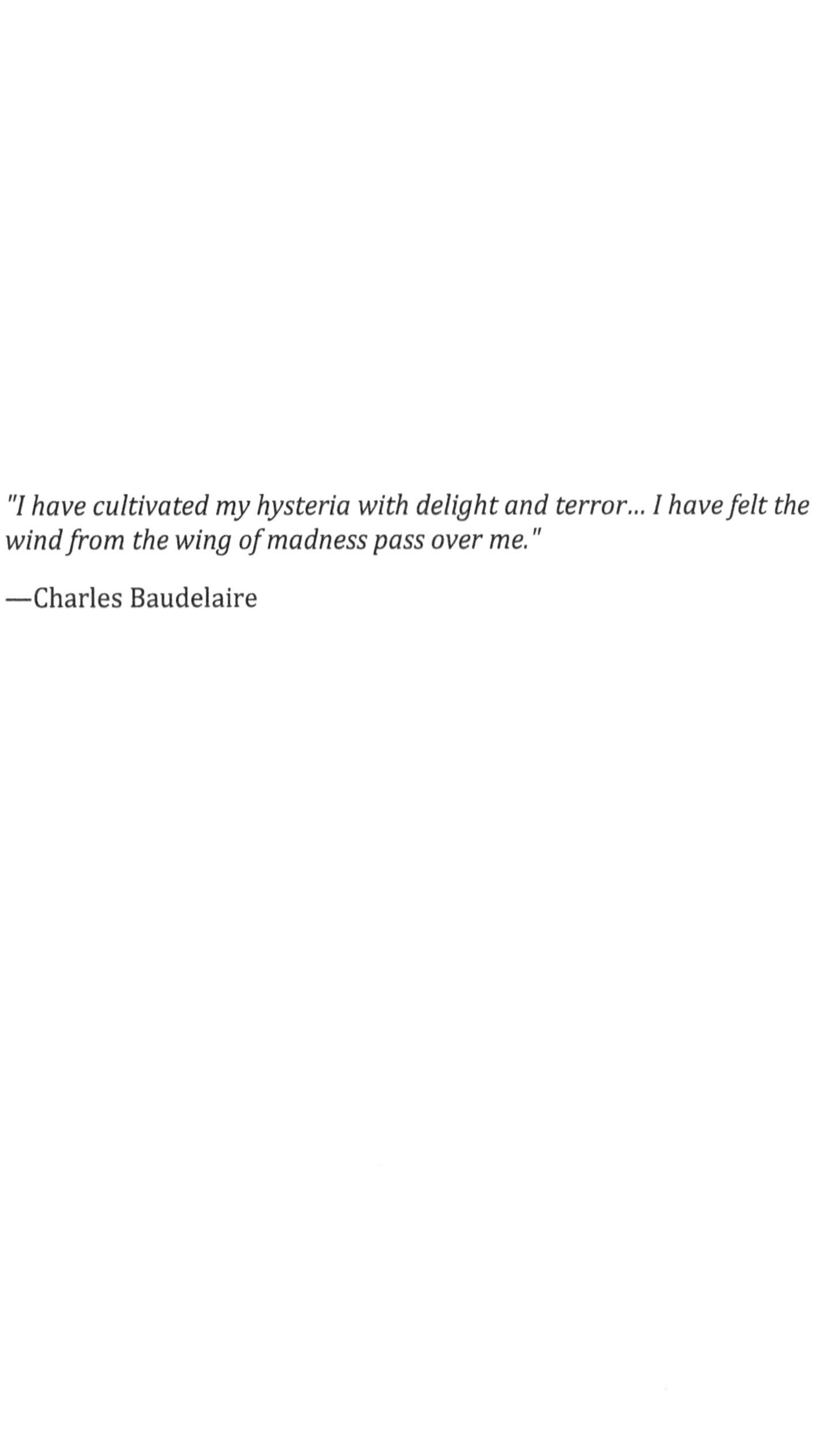

"I have cultivated my hysteria with delight and terror... I have felt the wind from the wing of madness pass over me."

—Charles Baudelaire

By December of 2013 I had finally had enough. All I had ever wanted was to just have a normal life, and I had done a decent job of making it look like I did. I was a 38-year-old mother of a brilliant 9-year-old son; I had been married to my high school sweetheart for almost 20 years; we had a beautiful home and successful careers; we were active church members; I was even managing to run five miles four to five times each week.

We looked really good, almost perfect, but it was all a cover up.

Nobody knew about the depression, anxiety and OCD that had followed me since childhood. My smile and my laugh kept me safe from the possibility of anyone ever knowing.

Nobody knew about the alcohol, the drugs or the endless arguing that went on behind closed doors. We were headed for divorce and had forgotten what love was.

Nobody knew about our desperate struggle to have more children. The miscarriages, the infertility and the enormous sense of loss were hidden from the outside world.

It was not until I started having suicidal thoughts that I sought professional help. I don't know why I waited so long other than I had always assumed that kind of help did not exist, but I had no other option. I was close to death. In the beginning I stayed alive for one reason: my son. I am grateful for that reason giving me the time I needed to begin healing and step onto my path of recovery. What a beautiful life I would have missed had I not chosen to get help!

The following are excerpts from the journals, prayers, poetry and emails I wrote. Yes, the experiences are uniquely mine, but they are also representative of the demons we all must face at some point in our lives. Welcome to the journey!

I.

Lost Soul

Year One: 2014

The Journey Begins

It happened very slowly; then, it happened all at once. The wind from the wing of madness brushed my face. It moved through my soul and stilled my beating heart as it carried me away to darkness and loneliness. Then the songs of angels echoed through my ears and delivered me to a world that placed me deep within my heart. I had to walk the path again through fire and through ice—up to heaven and down to hell, but to this day I don't remember if God pushed me or if I fell.

It is not that I cannot remember anything although there is obviously much I have forgotten. It is that the words simply do not exist to describe my emotions. None of them are good enough, and I have realized there are emotions which have been left un-named.

There is no word to describe the feeling that combines both the perfect harmony and the relentless despair felt when one stands at the point where heaven and hell intersect and manage to coexist...where leaving one means leaving the other and keeping one means keeping the other. There is also no word to identify how it feels to be in a prison with no walls where there is but one impossible requirement for freedom—the ability to just walk away.

No matter how far I have fallen, there is always a speck of light as the dust clears and I look up to where the sky should be. It takes time to ascend the unstable cliffs, but it can be done. There are many who are willing to help me along the way. They boost me up with their hands, let me stand on their shoulders, and throw me a rope. Some are even willing to climb down and sit with me right where I am until I am ready to climb. I know I cannot be carried out, but there are people who can help show me the way.

Letter To My Husband

Jack-

To love you or not to love you—that is the question. You were assigned the task of loving me, and you said you would, and you said you do—but how can I love you? I am afraid you will get better and I will still not be able to love you in the way I long for...to really connect and trust and know that you will catch me when I fall.

I remember the first time our eyes met. That time when you saw me and I saw you and we began this dance. No sparks and no flames. It was not love at first sight. We became *one* at first sight. Just peace and surrender. Is it possible to recognize someone you have never seen?

Perhaps we had never been anything but one. Our separateness an illusion of this world and this life. Two sides of the same coin who had never come face to face. Even if we had tried, neither of us would have been capable of breaking the magnetic pull of chaos to rigidity.

In the point midway between your gaze and mine, we sensed eternity, and we smiled. Juxtaposed hearts and mirror images of each other's souls. We found completeness. Two souls, exactly the same, would not match when put together face to face. They must be opposite in every detail to be placed together in a perfect overlay. Your strengths are my weakness. Your weaknesses are my strengths.

Since that first day, we have loved as much as we have hated. We have built each other up as much as we have torn each other down. We have served mightily for the Lord. You are an amazing father to our son, Grant. You always show up—but it is not enough. I need to know that you will catch me. I need to know that you won't be the one who has pushed me only to run to the bottom of the cliff and appear to rescue me. I love you and I want you to be the one, but I don't know how. You must release your demons too!

How can I reconcile two mutually exclusive worlds? A hateful love and an unconditional love? Both cannot exist in the same marriage. I suppose I can recognize, acknowledge, and bury the hateful love, but it must be put to rest. I need to know that it is dead.

Love,
Michelle

What It Feels Like When Heaven and Earth Collide

On the surface it begins like every other moment that has ever begun: normal, mundane, unextraordinary. The earth spins happily unaware of the struggles of its occupants and unconcerned by its own fragility. Time flies by as fleeting, but connected, moments.

Everything is as it should be: perfect harmony

Then, there is a slight wobble. The earth has lost its balance and begins to career wildly around like a spinning top headed for the edge of the table—moments and millimeters from an epic fall.

The moment suddenly becomes eternity. It is no longer connected to any other moment. It no longer exists in the realm of space and time because the world has violently exploded into tiny shards of glass. It is like lightning in its suddenness and shocking ability to disable. Everything stops. It is simply, but overwhelmingly, shocking. It is earth-shattering.

This is not how it should be: unrelenting despair

The world ceases to turn. There is only this moment. It contains everything. There is no pain, and there is no fear as the dreams pop one by one by one in rapid succession and the world goes fuzzy and I am no longer in it.

I am no longer in it. I am simply an observer of a shocking, eternal moment that plays endlessly and mercilessly over and over like a silent movie in my mind. Sound would make it impossible… unbearable, and so, it fades away moment by moment screaming silently into oblivion: forgotten and unknown.

Then, the world finds its balance and begins to turn again. It has not gone over the edge. It has not shattered beyond repair. It spins happily unaware of the struggles of its occupants and unconcerned by its own fragility.

Everything is as it should be: perfect harmony.

OCD

Yes, OCD has caused me to feel alone and embarrassed, but the loneliness and the shame have been the easy part.

Crushing in its overwhelming ability to severely oppress free will or choice, OCD subdues the soul by slowly grinding it into a fine powder—extracting all the remnants of hope and destroying all other options.

OCD makes itself the only option. There is no choice to make because there are no other options from which to choose.

The loss felt is incalculable—countless, immeasurable, and infinite. The value of life cannot be overestimated and life is certainly at stake.

The grief felt is limitless—sorrow and distress causing unimaginable suffering. The power of death cannot be overstated and death is surely imminent.

Pressed between reality and delusion the soul is broken.

Worshipping the Silence

Don't speak—maybe it will go away
Silence is sacred to secret scars
Don't speak—maybe you can really stay
Silence is sacred like wishes on stars

Keep it hidden—It's a private matter
Silence is sacred to buried screams
Keep it hidden—it's just an earth shatter
Silence is sacred—especially in dreams

Don't tell a soul—because, after all
Silence is sacred and must be respected
Don't tell a soul—what caused you to fall
Silence is sacred—leaving things undetected

Hush, hush—you mustn't cry
Silence is sacred in times of pain
Hush, hush—you don't want to die
Silence is sacred when there is rain

Don't pray to your God—He won't hear a thing
Silence is sacred to Satan's men
Don't pray to your God—He is only a King
Silence is sacred in the Serpent's den

Good morning Pastor Smith—

We met last year at the Christian Youth Conference in Colorado. You attended the seminar I was teaching on spiritual warfare, and we spoke several times over the next few days on topics such as depression, anxiety, and even the idea of my husband attending seminary. I have found that the Lord often puts people we need in our path; however, through our sinful nature, we often don't notice. I was really struggling at the time I met you last year and I should have contacted you then, but I didn't. Since I was a teenager, I have struggled with panic attacks, OCD, generalized anxiety, and depression. I went through most of my adult life as an atheist until the Lord placed me at the doorstep of St. Joseph's Church in Sacramento in 2007. It was there where I began to recover from much of my mental distress. I began to work diligently for the Lord and prayed for discernment in determining His will in my life. I went on mission trips to Ghana and began working as a youth group leader. I was filled with the Holy Spirit.

Somewhere along the way I stumbled. My panic attacks returned full force during a mission trip to Ghana in 2012 and during my trip with the youth group to Colorado. I began to lose faith and turned to my old friend who always patiently waits in the shadows for me to return: drugs. Needless to say, my life quickly spun out of control, and by the end of 2013, I was having intrusive and constant suicidal thoughts. I sought help through a Christian therapist who specializes in OCD and anxiety, but she quickly informed me of my substance abuse problem and redirected me to another therapist (a non-Christian therapist named Rachael). Through medication, prayer, and therapy I have now been in recovery for almost eight months (with the exception of a short relapse); however, it is only recently that I have been free of the suicidal thoughts.

Please do not be concerned with my safety. I would not place that burden on you, and I am in a healthy frame of mind with many people supporting me. I am also at the point where I am beginning to question how I can reconcile where I have been with being a

Christian. Is there a way to remain in therapy while maintaining a Christian worldview?

Is it possible to surrender my life to God and rely fully on Him while taking medication and going to therapy, or do the two contradict each other? How can a faithful Christian have succumbed to anxiety and depression?

I have been hesitant to blame my struggles on spiritual warfare or Satan's will, but I'm sure there is some of that occurring. I need your help and guidance in this battle. I have heard you are a battle-tested warrior! I was cleaning out my desk the other day and found my brochure from the youth conference. Your email and phone number were the only ones on the back of it. This time I could not ignore the fact that the Lord had placed you in my life for a reason. I would appreciate your prayers and advice.

Thank you,
Michelle

Pieces of Me—The Merge

The Vibrant Leader—a mirror to your soul. She is intelligent, confident, and strikingly familiar. The person you have always wanted to meet, and in whom you see a part of yourself, stands before you looking you straight in the eye. She is knowledgeable, passionate, and daringly bold. The teacher you have always wanted to have who helps you forge a new path in your head…and your heart…holds your hand as you prepare to move forward. She is articulate, eloquent and movingly spoken. The speaker you have always wanted to see who says the things you have always longed to hear is taking the stage.

The Faithful Worshipper—a carrier of hope. She is white-hot and on fire with the Holy Spirit. The Christian you have always hoped really exists walks into your life. She is brave and courageous—a risk taking soldier for the Lord. The warrior you want fighting on your side, who would lay down this temporary life in order to save your eternal one, shields you with the Lord's greatest weapon: LOVE. She is a compassionate, never-tiring servant. The missionary you pray knocks on the door of your mud hut…in your town without water or food or electricity to bring a spark of hope to your darkness…has arrived.

The Family Member—a wife, a mother, a daughter. She is devoted, understanding, and loving. The mother you wish were yours holds you and kisses you as she wipes away the tears. She is inadequate, unpredictable, and shockingly explosive. The mother you wish were dead crushes you with words. She is committed and faithful. The wife you want as your partner in life lies by your side and caresses your soul as you dream. She is hateful and unforgiving. The wife you should leave, but are afraid to let go of, begins to walk out the door yet never makes it out of the hallway. She is perfect and successful. A fake daughter you will never really know who stands like a porcelain doll on your shelf—beautiful yet so easily broken.

The Friend—a confidante and comrade. She is funny and uplifting and causes you to understand what C.S. Lewis meant when he said, "The typical expression of opening friendship would be something like, 'What? You too? I thought I was the only one." Someone who can always make you smile as you walk together down a secret path known only to the two of you. She is deeply connected yet always keeps you at an arm's length. You discover the friend you've been searching for is trapped behind a plate of glass as you reach in for a hug. Don't get too close to her heart. You might make it skip a beat...you might make it care.

The Shadow—a glimmer of a human being. She is frozen, afraid, and desperately alone. Unable to speak, the suicide you never noticed, or could never force yourself to watch, weeps silently. She is weak, trembling, and hoping it will all go away. Like a shadow, flickering in and out of the rays of sunlight, cowering in the dimly lit hallway of an abandoned building, she is sad and hopeless in her ignorance and isolation. A stumbler, unable to find the light switch or the door, who finally escapes into the daybreak only to fall to the ground for the last time beaten and burned into nothingness by the violent, unforgiving sun as she realizes <u>she cannot survive being exposed</u>.

The Writer—a muse to your life. She is open and honest as the words flow freely from her fingers. There are no barriers to what she might say. Someone who will say the things the world needs to hear, but she just can't speak, is shouting through the megaphone of the page. She knows the Leader, the Worshipper, the Family Member, the Friend, and even the Shadow. She recognizes and accepts them all as essential parts of herself. The have helped her survive. They have helped her thrive. The writer is nothing without the brilliant light and even less without the smothering darkness. She is capable of being white-hot and stone-cold in the same moment because she knows the two are necessary to maintain balance and truth in her life.

The Loser—a stoner lost in time. She has her feet kicked up on the couch and can hang with anyone. The partier you have always wanted to laugh with, who knows how to work hard and play hard, sits on the floor as she rolls one up on your coffee table. She is cool and relaxed as she blazes through life, yet she, like the Writer, knows and accepts all the others. She knows them because she is *all of them all the time.* She feels and moves to the rhythm of life, and recognizes the oneness of the world and the eternal moment that is now. She is careless and couldn't care less. It is all good as she dissolves into creation and her edges soften.

Double-edged Dagger

A ray comes shining in to pierce my heart. It is the hope of love. The hope of peace. The hope of completeness. It is now and only now. A ray that pierces the darkness and tears it to shreds.

Drugs are a double-edged dagger that cuts equally both ways. The more pain is all the more pleasure. Ecstasy and horror perch on the razor-sharp edges dripping with life...dripping with death. The more pleasure is all the more pain. I smile as the blade sinks deeper into my soul. Into my mind...until the searing pain cuts through to my core...and I smile and I cry behind blank eyes.

I would not say goodbye...because goodbye is too hard. I would just go.

Rachael—

I have decided it is probably not a good idea to wait until we are both geriatric patients to really allow you into my inner circle. My OCD takes many forms, some of which I was not aware of until very recently. As I've explored ways to deal with OCD, I've discovered I have been struggling with sexual OCD and homosexual OCD ever since I was a teenager. Making eye contact is often the equivalent to having a sexual encounter for me. Touching is even worse. I have intrusive thoughts regarding children, animals and homosexuality. The strange part is that I am actually very comfortable with my sexuality. It is one of the few areas in which my husband and I excel. I know who I am and what I enjoy. I am not gay. I do not want to have sex with animals. I would never sexually abuse my child. Needless to say, avoidance has been the way I deal with this problem. I avoid people and things that trigger my thoughts. Although the medication helps, I constantly remind and reassure myself that these things are not true, and I avoid any topic that is directly, or even indirectly, related to sex.

It is the reason I can't talk about our struggles with infertility and pregnancy loss.

It is the reason I've had a hard time talking about my relationship with my husband.

It is the reason I didn't want to discuss my issues with the antidepressants.

When you asked me yesterday what my life without anxiety would look like, I gave you a very concrete example; however, I think that often the abstract is much more real and truthful than the tangible. The abstract delivers an experience and an emotional response unlike a simple example from this world that is quickly passing away. You have used the term "old soul" a few times, and as uncomfortable as the term makes me feel, I think it is fitting here. I always thought it would be amazing to be an old soul as it conjured up images of wisdom and understanding; however, I have come to experience it as being nothing less than a curse that leaves one weary of the world and the life it offers. If I had to bet, I'd say you probably run across many of these people in your line of work. This is my truth and this is what it would look like if there were no anxiety in my life. Thank you for being the person I can share this with. I have carried it alone for a very long time, and I am eternally grateful the Lord placed you in my path.

Fearless Old Souls
(or What an Anxiety-free Life Would Look Like)

It would look like two old souls suddenly crossing each other's paths once again as they wait at an intersection of life. Finding themselves face-to-face, they find no need to nod or wink because the recognition is instantaneous. Their eyes meet and smile a thousand smiles at the remembrance of a thousand lifetimes gone by and the knowledge of the eternal life that is now. As they become one with each other and the world they occupy, they feel the earth heave a deep and joyous sigh of hope as it is freed from the weight of itself and allows the moon to move its waters and the sun to warm its beaches. They dance in and out with the tides and are carried by the moonbeams on the water as they engage in an endless and fearless embrace and their hearts become one. Love flows simply and naturally from everlasting springs and falls like perfectly unique snowflakes onto their tongues, and they are refreshed and renewed. They are ready to move on. They are able to let go. They release their gazes and continue walking knowing they are always headed home no matter where they stand.

Amazing Grace

No longer need to run
Nor struggle to race with the sun
Afraid of what the night brings.

Darkness—it is my greatest fear
For that is when evil begins to draw near
While Satan quietly sings.

Tying my mind in endless knots
While my beautiful heart—it simply rots
As he whispers of terrible things.

Claiming to be my one true friend
He says to hell I must descend
To escape and earn my wings.

A gun to my head or a pill to my lips
I'd never again feel God's fingertips
As His call—it endlessly rings.

The Father of Lies—he fills my head
With the promise of freedom when I am dead
My soul he shrewdly flings.

His hell is not hot, nor is it bright
But is bitter cold and absent of light
As I say my goodbye, his searing gaze stings.

No more need to listen to the dark voice
I clearly see that I have a choice
To return to my King of Kings.

Welcoming me back to the Word that saves
Not scared of the dark—not scared of the graves
With the hope and the love His grace brings.

Letter to my Son

*The so-called 'psychotically depressed' person who tries
to kill herself doesn't do so out of quote 'hopelessness' or
any abstract conviction that life's assets and debits do
not square. And surely not because death seems
suddenly appealing. The person in whom an invisible
agony reaches a certain unendurable level will kill
herself the same way a trapped person will eventually
jump from the window of a burning high-rise. Make no
mistake about people who leap from burning windows.
Their terror of falling from a great height is still just as
great as it would be for you or me standing
speculatively at the same window just checking out the
view; i.e. the fear of falling remains a constant. The
variable here is the other terror, the fire's flames. And
yet nobody down on the sidewalk, looking up and
yelling 'Don't!' and 'Hang on!' can understand the jump.
Not really. You'd have to have personally been trapped
and felt flames to really understand a terror way
beyond falling.—David Foster Wallace*

Dear Grant-

I want you to know what I have done so I could be with you today:

I have stood on the window's ledge of a building engulfed in an
inferno of the mind, and I have felt the heat of the flames flickering
at my feet encouraging me to jump, and I have turned around to face
my demons.

I did this so you will be able to fights yours, too.

I have fallen into the fiery oceans of hell that turned my breath to ashes, and I have fought the desire to surrender to the current's pull as the shore quickly faded away, and I have kept swimming.

I did this so you could sing that song while you refuse to look at my camera instead of searching the audience for a mother who no longer exists.

I have battled monsters that have carried me into the abyss of my heart, and I have clawed my way out of that deep, dark place, and I have slain the dragon that circled around patiently waiting for me to fall.

I did this so you can laugh that beautiful laugh in the face of danger as you remember that you come from a long line of dragon slayers.

I have lived with a frozen heart that has been shattered many times, and I have picked up its jagged pieces as they cut deeply into my hands, and I have put it painstakingly back together.

I did this so I could love you just one more time...and then once more.

I have clung to the thread of hope that hangs from the Lord's glorious robes, and I have begged Him to remove the thorn of anxiety, and I have learned that His grace IS enough for me.

I did this so you can pray that prayer for a guinea pig instead of the prayer for my return, and I will do it again tomorrow so I can be with you today.

Love,
Mom

Reflection

As the year comes to a close, I am forced to reflect on all that has happened. The year was almost a total loss and failure due to my complete surrender to panic, anxiety, fear, depression and suicidal thoughts. At the start of the year, I was not quite sure when I had stepped off the path of faith and eternal happiness and onto the path of hopelessness and into the abyss of eternal despair. I am now beginning to see that much of it began as I realized my hope of having another child would never materialize. Perhaps it was also when our seventeen-year-old nephew, Ray, moved in a few years ago and became both a testament to the power of the Holy Spirit and a massive test of my own faith. As strange as it might seem, I think I lost my way while on my second mission trip to Ghana. The panic and fear that suddenly reappeared after years of peace changed the course of my life and eventually led to my current struggle. As the year Ray lived with us was a testament to the power of the Holy Spirit, this year of my life has been a testament to the power of the devil and the severe inadequacies of the human heart and will. I refuse to allow this to continue!

II.

Naked Soul

Year Two: 2015

Making Progress

I have come a very long way, yet I have an eternal distance ahead of me. I have read that the journey of a thousand miles begins with the first step. Last year was that first step for me. I now find myself awakened to a new life—a life built by my old self, including many good and many bad choices. It is a life that has been here all the while, but I was never able to experience it because I was always running and hiding from the parts of it that scared me—the parts of it that hurt. I have discovered that, to enjoy the pleasure, I must endure the pain and sometimes the pain opens doors that can never be opened when I am comfortable.

Doors that have opened from the pain of the first step of my journey:

- Deeper faith, understanding, and love of God
- Patience
- Friendship—real friendship
- Trust—in myself and others
- Better communication
- A voice—I no longer suffer in silence—I can speak the unspeakable
- A quiet, peaceful mind
- LOVE—in all areas of my life

Liquid Horizon

The Lord calls me by name as the sun sets on the liquid horizon and is gently absorbed and the waves crash along the well-armed shoreline in a battle of life and death for a place in this world. Chaos and calm balanced in the frame of this eternal moment remind me of the many sunsets of my soul as I am absorbed and engulfed by the Lord's love after the violent struggles for a place in His house.

Lies the Devil Told Me
(The Lies My Fantasy World Supports)

- I will never get better because therapy never works and medications are a scam of the big pharma companies
- I will eventually die by suicide because I am hopelessly trapped
- I do not have a substance abuse problem—it is only anxiety and OCD
- All people are inconsistent, untrustworthy, and unreliable
- I am using people or wasting their time if they are fulfilling some kind of need for me
- People do not really care about or want to help me
- My family is too self-centered to care or understand my problems
- OCD compulsions will keep bad things from happening
- Drugs will help my anxiety, insomnia, depression, and social anxiety
- I have permanently damaged Grant with my behavior and he will have mental health problems as an adult and will never have a happy marriage
- God abandoned me when I turned my back on Him
- I can never find any long term happiness
- If I want something done, I should do it myself—I do not need or like other people
- If I admit to loving or needing someone, they will see it as inappropriate and they will abandon me
- I am a bad mother
- I am a bad person
- I do not have enough faith
- All therapists/psychiatrists are crazy
- Medication will make me a zombie
- I will never have a close relationship with my family members
- My depression and anxiety are my identity
- I will never be able to travel

- Nobody has a "normal," non-chaotic life—all families are dysfunctional
- My miscarried children are not real and I need to move on and forget about them—they were only dreams
- My Christian friends will not understand my drug problem or my suicidal thoughts, so I should not share my story with them
- I do not need to grieve for the loss of "hoped for" children
- I am incapable of having or properly caring for another child
- We should not consider adoption
- I can't do this—I should give up

Infinite Joy and Infinite Sorrow

Yesterday I went to my first circular breathing meditation. It was nothing short of what I would imagine a walk with God might feel like. I felt intense joy and love while at the same time feeling deep sorrow at the separation I have always felt from this Love that has always been there.

Behold, the Kingdom of God is within you—Luke 17:21

The Cup of Life

Bitter sweet the first few sips
As I place the metal to my lips
My head begins to spin with fear
For death is indisputably near
As I begin to drink and my heart skips

Growing more accustomed to the taste
I realize I had judged in haste
The fluid begins to fill my soul
And cleanse my heart that has gone dull
With years of seeing love as waste

No more days filled with strife
For once—safe from the knife
That cuts deep to the core
Asking what's it all for?
Exchanging death for the cup of life

Hello from Heaven

Last night I went to my second breathing meditation class. It was the most beautiful, intense experience I have ever had. Nothing compares to it. Last night, as I focused on my breath, my mind was free to release what it had held away to keep me safe. Last night, as I became a flower floating on the river, I found my lost children playing along the riverbank. I noticed them before they noticed me. They were holding hands and laughing and dancing as they played in the presence of God. When they saw me, they calmly and gently came over to me and helped me onto the shore. There were no words spoken because there was no need. Everything was perfectly understood. I have never allowed myself to acknowledge them—yet here they stood. They were beautiful and the age they would be today if they walked the earth. Without speaking I told them I loved them and they told me they loved me.

These children of God each gave me a flower that looked like a daisy—brown center with deep orange petals. Then they returned me to the river and I floated home. As I wept during meditation, I allowed myself to be held. I allowed my forehead to be caressed. I allowed a teardrop to gently fall onto the finger of a new friend who has been placed by the Lord in my path. I allowed myself to receive the love and nurturing of a caring woman who was willing to sit with me in my pain—willing to feel it with me—willing to breathe for me when the emotions were too overwhelming. I was safe.

Your Father knows what you need before you ask Him—Matthew 6:8

The True Author

It is ironic that suicidal thoughts are what saved my life and changed my trajectory. Sometimes God allows terrible things into our lives to serve a purpose: His purpose. The Lord allowed Satan to approach me face to face and heart to heart. I could see and feel all of his empty promises—empty hopes—empty solutions. God allowed Satan to weaken me because, when I am weak, then I am strong.

I will hand the authorship of my life to its true narrator—God. I am a terrible author who apparently cannot think of any new or creative endings to my story. I'm sure the Lord has something in mind. Lord—please help me—please be the author again. –Amen

Adoption Decision Letter

Rachael-

Jack and I have decided to move forward with the process of adoption from foster care. I am very aware of the risks associated with adoption, and it is something we have given an extraordinary amount of thought to over several years. Obviously, adopting a newborn would minimize the risks and losses inherent in adoption; however, we are not, nor have we ever been, comfortable with the idea of paying large amounts of money and competing with a long line of people in order to, what I think amounts to, purchase an "undamaged" white newborn. We have always wanted to enlarge our family by at least one more child, and we have explored many options, and we have been patient despite my apparent lack of patience in general. The process of adopting from foster care generally takes 1-2 years, so we feel the time is right to begin now even though I am still struggling with my anxiety. I am very comfortable with the idea of adopting and have never had an issue with being able to accept a non-biological child as my own. However, there are two areas in which I am uncomfortable: 1) By committing to adoption I am acknowledging a great loss along with a great longing in my life and 2) I am concerned with how I believe people will respond.

I am pretty sure I realized I wanted to move forward with this after the breathing meditation experiences I had. Being able to recognize my grief helped me to see which direction I think is best for me and my family. I am confronted with my loss/inability to have another child on a daily basis. When Corrinne mentions during our women's group she has no one to help with her mother because she is an only child, I am reminded the same is true of Grant. When my son realizes and tells me he will never be an uncle, I am reminded of what an amazing brother I know he would be. When I refer to the kid and not the kids, I am reminded that society easily and readily accepts the phrase the boys, but cringes at and does not accept "the boy." I can accept my physiological inability to have another child; however, I cannot accept simply sitting back and allowing an opportunity to pass.

I have been hesitant to discuss this issue with you because I know you have seen the negative side of adoption in many of your clients. I am very aware that an adopted child has suffered incredible loss and has life-long issues relating to early childhood trauma and neglect. I consider adoption to be the intersection of two tragic paths that, not without great effort, carries the hope of healing and love in the midst of pain, loss, and struggles. I'm also sure you have doubts regarding my "stability," but I can assure you I deal quite well with real obstacles. Pretend obstacles that are all in my head are another story.

Naked Soul

Naked soul exposed to the light
Peeks through each cut of the knife
Before it begins to cry

Naked soul exposed to the night
Weaves through each thread of life
Before it begins to die

Naked soul exposed to the sun
Twists through each grueling day
Before it begins to fry

Naked soul exposed on the run
Looks through to find a way
Before it begins to try

Naked soul exposed under cover
Trembles through each passing storm
Before it begins to dry

Naked soul exposed by a lover
Shivers through an embrace so warm
Before it begins to sigh

Naked soul exposed by the path it travels
Walks through to the other side
Before it begins to ask why

Naked soul exposed as the lie unravels
Sees through and starts to confide
Before it begins to fly

Naked soul exposed as the truth
Surrenders through the revealing
Before it begins to reach for the sky

Naked soul exposed as uncouth
Passes through the need for concealing
Before it begins to end the lie

Rachael—

OK, so I feel like sharing and decided I would fill you in on some of the blanks you have due to my not sending you any journals over the past few months. It looks like you didn't entirely miss that window of opportunity. You really should have pushed me more today to send you some journals. Ha, ha, just kidding!

On a more serious note, this February I had another miscarriage. No matter how many times it has happened and regardless of whether we are still "trying to conceive," it always spins my mind. Sorry I didn't share, but it is extremely personal and I relied on my old way of dealing with things on my own. I wrote this journal shortly after my second breathing meditation in March. It is really a combination of me coming to terms with my losses while at the same time acknowledging the gifts the Lord has blessed me with. The children in my journal do represent my actual losses; however, they are also reflections of some of the "lost" parts of myself.

A Meditation and a Prayer

Breathe in. Breathe out. Let go—open—the heart—the mind.
The Holy Spirit pours out infinite love and fills me beyond earthly limitations.

The pain is set free as I feel the atonement and behold the Kingdom of God that is within me. I am safe. I am free. The infinite sorrow escapes the clutches of my heart...

Cradled in the arms of Love. Perfect joy. Perfect peace.

Floating along the current of the river in the presence of God. The sweet, soft sound of His voice brings comfort, and His words remind me that, although Satan hates me, my Father loves me much, much more.

Once a slave to sin, I am now a slave to perfect Love as I see who I was truly meant to be.

In my surrender I can see the edge of heaven, and I can watch the horizon where the sun is always rising...its light bringing a soft glow to anything and anyone it touches. In my surrender I can see it is at heaven's edge where God's children come to play...and they are holding hands along the riverbank.

The first child: Peaceful Love
A nurturer who knows no worries or fears because she has felt perfect love and perfect love is something that can never be fully forgotten. She is free to comfort all who come to her, so she approaches me with a flower and wipes away my tears.

Lord, you created me as a loving and caring person, but the world has led me to believe that I must be cold and heartless. Lord, with your help, I will comfort those you send to me.

The second child: Silent Sage
He is a guide to hold the hands of children and show them to the riches that await them. Full of the knowledge of God's grace, he stands calmly pointing the way for me with one hand while clutching a flower in the other.

Lord, you covered me with your grace and pointed me in the direction of heaven, but the world has made me question your trustworthiness. Are you who you claim to be? Lord, with your help, I will guide your children back to you.

The third child: Joyous Delight
A playful child held down by nothing because there is no reason to be concerned as he is being bathed in the glow of the rising sun, and feeling the need to share his delight, he approaches me with a flower.

Lord, you created me as a joyful and delighted child, but the world has made me hopeless and sad. Lord, with your help, I will bring your joy back into the lives of the people you place in my path.

The fourth child: Innocent Purity
He is the one still too small to travel to heaven's edge to play, so he is rocked gently to sleep in the arms of the Lord. He is afraid of nothing—innocently fearless—sinless. He is unaware of the flower resting gently on his chest as he breathes the weightless breaths of sleep.

Lord, you formed me from the beginning as an innocent child, but the world has turned me into a scared and sinful adult. Lord, with your help, I will be fearless with the hope you have given me by making me sinless in your presence.

--Amen

Rachael—

It is true that sometimes I give you 0%, but it is also true that sometimes I give you 100%. This is one of those occasions. Keep in mind that this journal is only representative of the sexual aspects of my OCD, but I think this is much more useful in uncovering why it is so difficult for me to bring down my wall with you.

It is not really about you personally, nor is it about sex specifically. It is about what you represent—a relationship I am starving for—one in which I allow myself the guidance of a safe female figure who I really trust.

The sexual aspect of this is simply a mechanism to dehumanize you. We live in a culture that is both hypersexual and sexually repressed, so there is great power in its symbolism. I have realized the OCD thoughts keep me from fully entering and navigating a complex relationship in which I must let go and risk falling into the abyss, yet at the same time, I stand to gain the possibility of "falling up." It is a huge gamble.

Sexual OCD

To soothe my own concerns, it is important for me to begin this with who I am because who I actually am, although far from normal or perfect, does not bother me. What bothers me is who I might unknowingly be, who I might become, or who others believe I am. I am a loving and compassionate mother who would do anything to protect my child, but sometimes I have a short temper and very little patience. I am a moody and difficult wife, but I love my husband and, despite our flaws, we make a pretty good team sometimes. Even though he is not a "safe" person, I am open with him, have a longstanding and healthy sexual relationship with him, and do not experience any OCD related to him. In fact, I have even shared some of my sexual OCD thoughts with him. In regards to sexuality: I believe it is outside the realm of morality (good or bad); I have no judgement towards people who are gay or bisexual; and I am comfortable with the fact that I am attracted to men while at the same time can acknowledge/recognize the beauty or sexual energy of women. I also believe sexuality can be fluid, is not set in stone, and most people fall into three main categories: mostly heterosexual, mostly homosexual, or bisexual. I think very few people are 100% sexually attracted to only one gender and are being dishonest if they deny it. Before moving forward, and in order to be more open with my OCD thoughts, it is important for me to clarify certain main points: 1) I am heterosexual 2) I am not sexually attracted to animals 3) I am not sexually attracted to children 4) I would never harm an animal or a child.

Sexual OCD has tormented me since I was a child. I have intrusive thoughts at the worst possible times. The first memories I have of obsessive sexual thoughts are around the age of 12 or 13. I was petting one of our cats and began to fear I was going to touch him in a sexual way. I became overwhelmed with worry that I might become attracted to animals, or I might be attracted and just not realize it, or someone might think that I was (even though I wasn't). I was also worried I would impulsively act on my thoughts. These thoughts and worries occurred when I was around my pets and also at times when I wasn't expecting them. They almost always occurred around animals that are not shy about covering up their "private areas." These thoughts sometimes involve graphic sexual images and I often avoid looking at animals out of fear that, if I look too long, it would mean my fears were true, or it would be noticed by others, or it would cause me to become aroused.

Over my teenage years these fears progressed to include more areas of sexuality. I began to fear that I would hurt a child, or if I looked too long at a child, it meant I would be inappropriately attracted to him or her. I began to fear that I would impulsively harm a child and began to avoid situations such as public pools and restrooms. I would also mentally check to make sure I was not sexually aroused in any way if a child was near. During this time, I also began to fear I would become gay even though I didn't think I was. I would look at pictures of men and women to make sure I was appropriately attracted to the men and not attracted to the women. If someone was in the room with me and I saw a picture or a show with a woman on it, I would have to look away in case someone noticed I was attracted to her (even though I wasn't). I also began to avoid places such as dressing rooms or school/gym locker rooms that involved changing clothes in public. I also worry when I am around someone who is gay because I fear he/she will either cause me to become gay or they will "know" I am gay even if I am not. The funny part of this is, if I truly were gay or bisexual, I would be ok with it. It's not something I would be ashamed of or try to hide. It's that I am not gay or bisexual that makes it so distressing.

Most of these obsessive thoughts have continued off and on throughout my life. The medication helps in that it weakens the strength of the thoughts, but I still have them on a daily basis. Now I am usually able to let them go; however, if I am very anxious, I will do what I need to do to avoid the thoughts such as leaving a situation or changing the subject. I will sometimes carefully choose my words in order to avoid saying anything that could be interpreted as sexual either directly or indirectly. I stay off the topic completely. A current example would be how I was so nervous about the first yoga class you had me try. Most of the reason for my anxiety can be blamed on the fear I had that there would be a public changing area I would need to use because it was "hot" yoga and would require changing out of sweat soaked clothes and, in my world, nakedness=sex. Additionally, yoga puts people in close proximity to one another and in very vulnerable positions. In my world, closeness=sex. I also continue to fear becoming attracted to or aroused by male animals, particularly my own. I also continue to make sure I don't look too long at children and avoid looking at or coming into contact with any area that could be perceived as sexually inappropriate. This is part of the reason surrounding my anxiety regarding the youth group trip to Colorado and living for a week in such a close environment. The only reason I am able to have a close relationship with Grant is because I constantly reassure myself that I know I would never hurt him and it is just my OCD. I have been able to let the thoughts go.

Over the years I have discovered ways I can avoid being in situations that trigger my unwanted thoughts. I know who or what types of people/situations generally trigger my thoughts. When I really love something or someone, the relationship becomes transformed into a twisted sexual thought. There immediately become zero degrees of separation between anything that person does/says/wears/etc. and sex. I experience graphic sexual images. Did I look too long? What if I impulsively hurt that child or that animal? I really admire that person. Does that mean I am gay? I have to look away.

Eye contact=sex
Physical contact=sex
Vulnerability=sex
Love=sex
Connection=sex
Respect and admiration=sex

Oscar Wilde once said, "Everything is about sex, except sex. Sex is about power." He was right. I'm not sure if this is really not all about power and control. When I feel like someone is weak or I can control them or how they see me, then I do not have the intrusive thoughts or the thoughts are very weak and much more manageable. That is also probably why I don't have these thoughts very often in relation to men. I think women generally hold a higher level of "real" power over men and are in control of most interactions. Don't ask why. It is just the way I feel. A very small and oversimplified example of this idea of control is when you shared with me that you had never really used drugs. It gave me more control in our relationship than I had before, and so I have had less intrusive thoughts surrounding our interactions. In my world, personal information about a person gives me control. That has been a large part of my problem with you. I understand the professional nature of our relationship, but it is also very difficult for me to really take part in a relationship that is so one-sided in who gets what information regarding the other.

I think it is pretty obvious why someone growing up with these thoughts would never discuss them with anyone; however, I have been very hesitant to discuss them with you because, as I'm sure you are aware, you are a very strong trigger for my OCD. There is an inherent uncomfortableness in all of this, but you asked me to give you an example, so I will make it personal. Keep in mind that I have this problem with any woman I consider to be strong, intelligent, funny, loving and attractive. This is basically a replica of many relationships I have had, so don't let it go to your head.

Basically everything about you causes me to doubt myself. Sounds pretty fucking gay to me except for the fact that I can't stand the thoughts I have. I want them to go away so I can just be myself (because the real me is super awesome ha, ha). The control and power you have over our interactions causes severely distressing thoughts for me. In my world, ALL relationships are about control and power and you have been much too squirrely to give me any of it. The only reason I have ever come back is because I know I need to get past these thoughts in order to truly be and stay in recovery. It is no wonder I turned to drugs to turn off my thoughts. Hope I didn't make you uncomfortable…ha, ha just kidding!

Peace,
Michelle

I shared with Rachael a few weeks back that I didn't consider my journal to be a story of great hope because the end has not been written yet, and it could end very badly. In my attempt at integration, I have found my journal IS a story of great hope precisely because of the fact that it has always swung from being a hopeless note to being a joyful, hopeful prayer. This journal is essentially snippets of both ends of the pendulum over the last 18 months. As a disclaimer, I would like to emphasize that I am NOT at the bad end of the spectrum right now. I'm hanging out somewhere in the middle.

Lost and Found

A life lost and found in a hopeless note
I stood on the ledge of a window's sill
I can't take anymore—is what I wrote
Growing tired of the search for God's will

A life lost and found in a hopeless note
I fought dragons that really were frogs
I must run towards them—is what I wrote
Killing with metaphorical logs

A mind lost and found in a hopeless note
I decided my death was my own
Goodbye my sweet boy—is what I wrote
Not thinking of when he was grown

A mind lost and found in a hopeless note
Not sure of what I would find
Fearless, old souls—is what I wrote
Walking through the labyrinth of my mind

A heart lost and found in a hopeless note
I was broken by sadness and shame
I'm afraid of love—is what I wrote
Finding my obsessive thoughts to blame

A heart lost and found in a hopeless note
Was healed by an unlikely crew
They sure seem real—is what I wrote
Now, what I am I to do?

A soul lost and found in a hopeless note
I was crushed by loss and pain
My God has abandoned me—is what I wrote
There is nothing left here to gain

A soul lost and found in a hopeless note
I found my "self" in the breath
I must return my life to the Lord—is what I wrote
The Author who steals life from death

One Year

One year ago this week I started to relapse. As I approach my one year of sobriety, I find myself not as impressed as I thought I would be. I have realized this is not a battle that is won in a year—nor is it a battle that can be won in a lifetime of years—nor does it really have anything to do with alcohol or drugs. It can only be won in the moment. The moment of temptation...moment of boredom... moment of fear...moment of desire...moment of yearning. The moment when I am face to face with God and the devil and must decide with whom I prefer to dance. There is always that choice, and it is always only in this moment. Not in a day. Not in a year.

I once wrote there is no word to describe what it is like to stand at the point where heaven and hell intersect and manage to coexist. I was wrong. That word is simply called life, and in this year I have found I must surrender to each moment as it arrives filled with its heavens and its hells—whether it is surrendering to the deep waters of sadness or surrendering to the ecstasy of the sunrise declaring the glory of God. One year amounts to a great deal of surrender. One year ago marks the beginning of my surrender. That is the thing to celebrate.

Rachael-

When you asked me today about what we did with Grant's old room, I totally gave you a "standard" answer. The truth is, I have allowed myself to be hopeful regarding the adoption process and the room is ready for whomever God decides to drop off at our doorstep, but it is particularly ready for a young child. Grant had a lot of stuff from when he was little, and he helped me put the room together. It was really nice to have that time and share that dream with him and also to allow myself to be hopeful about the future. It is really difficult for me to express how I feel, but I can say it brings tears to my eyes to think about it. Not sure if they are happy or sad tears. Probably both.

Lately, I have really felt a lot of things coming together in a meaningful way.

Synchronicity

A falling together in space and time—my life becomes yours and yours becomes mine. Some call it chance, but I, I call it divine when the Lord places me in your path and you in mine. There is no explanation as to why; there is only a smile from the hazy, blue sky.

There is no such thing as chance when the Lord speaks and the angels dance as our souls intertwine at the intersection of your path and mine. When the heavens wink and say, "Remember, I am with you always, but especially today," I can no longer ignore that I am part of a whole, I am one with humanity; I am not a separate soul.

Satan weeps when the earth whispers my name, when I can see God's power, and the Lord's plan becomes clear in a simple, orange flower. We spin together for no cause, no effect, as our lives, once separate, will now always connect. A reminder of the joy I may truly find when I seek the innocence and purity so long ago left behind.

A falling together in space and time—my life becomes yours and yours becomes mine. Two separate paths become one as we are gently reminded there is nothing new under the sun. The Lord places peace in my mind as we fall together in space and time and the angels dance to a tune divine.

Youth Conference Seminar

Rachael-

Nice work today sticking with your line of questioning despite my diversion tactics. Sorry, but I hadn't planned on talking about the topic of my workshop for the upcoming Colorado Youth Conference and I hadn't really thought it through all the way. I don't like talking about things that have not been fully developed and perfected in my head, especially if they are very important to me. I also get very uncomfortable when my soul is showing which happens when I discuss my faith or any other important thing that actually causes me to feel a strong emotion. Remember, I am just as uncomfortable sharing very positive feelings as I am showing negative ones. The connection is just too much sometimes. Here is what I will be covering at this year's conference:

"Spiritual Warfare: Claiming Victory in Jesus Christ When Things Seem Hopeless."

In my workshop I will be focusing on 2 Corinthians 12:7-10

Therefore, in order to keep me from becoming conceited, I was given a thorn in my flesh, a messenger of Satan, to torment me. Three times I pleaded with the Lord to take it away from me. But he said to me, "My grace is sufficient for you, for my power is made perfect in weakness." Therefore I will boast all the more gladly about my weaknesses, so that Christ's power may rest on me. That is why, for Christ's sake, I delight in weaknesses, in insults, in hardships, in persecutions, in difficulties. <u>For when I am weak, then I am strong</u>.

God's grace gives us hope and healing in a world filled with suffering and temptation. Through personal examples I will demonstrate how the Holy Spirit is with us at every point of temptation and will come to us even in the depths of despair and weakness to walk with us. I hope to share my pain in a way the youth will understand:

The pain of addiction
The pain of shame
The pain of anxiety, depression, and OCD
The pain of isolation
The pain of seeking perfection in a fallen world

I also plan to share with them the lies the devil spoke to me as I fell away from my faith:

The lie that it will never get better
The lie that there is nobody in this world who can be trusted or who cares about me
The lie that a person of faith could never end up where I was
The lie that I must remain silent
The lie that death and eternal separation from God was the only way to end my pain

There will also be a worksheet for the youth to explore their own areas of suffering and temptation and how those circumstances can either build their faith or cause them to turn away from God. I plan to share the ways in which my struggles caused me to abandon my faith, and ultimately, regain a stronger faith and relationship with God. I might even mention the people He put in my path to help and how those relationships have helped me! I might even share a couple of my journals! Maybe.

Meditation with God

Do not let your hearts be troubled. You believe in God; believe also in me. My Father's house has many rooms; if that were not so, would I have told you that I am going there to prepare a place for you? And if I go and prepare a place for you, I will come back and take you to be with me that you also may be where I am. You know the way to the place where I am going—John 14:1-5

I went to my third breathing meditation last night. As is now becoming a pattern, it was nothing short of a conversation and encounter with God. I asked for more surrender to His will in my life and I asked Him what He wants from me. God came to me and showed me that the room in His house He is preparing for me has always been there. We stood at the center of my heart. God has been preparing my heart so I might dwell in love for eternity.

He gave me the vision of Christ crucified and I became one with Christ on the cross. My hands and feet were nailed to it, and a crown of thorns was placed by God's very hands onto my head releasing a blinding light from each puncture into my skin. He said <u>He wants nothing less than all of me</u>. He wants my life. He wants me to be Christ crucified so I might love the world and His creation as He does. To be Christ crucified I must lay down my sins at the feet of the cross and I must suffer as Christ did for me. I must experience the thirst and the mockery and the sponge of vinegar on my lips. I must hang from the cross and ask, "My God, My God—why have you forsaken me?" I must be pierced through to the inner sanctuary of my heart pouring out every last ounce of life giving blood in my soul—and my sky must turn black.

Only when I experience Christ crucified can I understand what He has done for me and what He wants me to do for others. He wants my love to flow over humanity so all may enter into the living water that is the source of life from the beginning to the end. God spoke to me and said, "I want you to bring me back my children for you know the way. Bring me my beautiful children whom I love so deeply.

Carry all your suffering to those who suffer. Carry your cross so others may see that it is possible. Carry with you all whom I have given you as guides. Turn your suffering and your sorrow into praise and joy because your suffering has crushed you enough to finally hear my voice."

Then He released me back onto the river and I heard a bell calling me home. It was a bell singing of the great hope that can only be found in the depths of suffering. It was in the depths of hell where the Lord waited patiently for me to take His hand and let Him lead me. Let Him carry me.

Let them prepare a sanctuary for me, that I may dwell among them—
Exodus 25:8-9

Do you not know that your body is a temple of the Holy Spirit who is in you, whom you have from God and you are not your own—
1Corinthians 6:19

Disconnected and Rejected

Disconnected and rejected becoming broken once again
Awakened from its dreaming state the world begins to spin
As it falls into the mortal gap that wanders by from time to time
It begins to break in half becoming pieces of yours and mine

Disconnected and rejected time does not end in fire or in ice
But in the subtle sadness of a distant lover's fading voice
That echoes through the mountains and in the deep and angry pride
Reflected by the endless battle between the moon and the ocean's
tide

Disconnected and rejected in the end there is no victory—no winner
But a bitter heart replaces love and serves a cold and lonely dinner
Ceaseless knocking at the door reveals the truth of no one here
When the world has been consumed by clouds of disdain and fear

Disconnected and rejected the end replaces the beginning
A memory turned inside out and upside down is quickly thinning
No more wishing on stars as the dream of completeness is now over
It was all a lie. It was all a lie. There's no such thing as four leaf
clovers

No! No! Wait! Wait! That can't possibly be all
There must be more to humanity than just the long and winding fall
If this is where the story ends, then this is where the devil wins
With all his deadly promises and all his heavenly sins

Connected and accepted the sun must set if it wishes to rise
And the earth continues spinning while embraced by cloudy skies
Bolts of lightning, cracks of thunder, and torrential bouts of rain
At first appearing deadly—but meant to wash away the pain

Connected and accepted standing face to face with the divine
There is suddenly no difference. There is no dividing line
Because in the brightest day there is a speck of furious night
And in the darkest evening there is a remnant of hopeful light

Connected and accepted there is no beginning. There is no end
A future hope once long forgotten can be seen beyond the bend
A path cleared in the flood of tears and quiet, gentle weeping
Leads to a place of truth and the harvest meant for reaping

Connected and accepted to a promise He once made
Providing comfort and protection in the valley filled with shade
Being led by still waters there is no need for anger or for fear
Lying down in His green pastures knowing He is always near

Adoption Social Worker

Rachael-

Yesterday we met our actual social worker, Katie, who will be completing the home study and helping to match us with a child. We really liked her and had no problem/uncomfortableness talking with her. So far we have not had anything other than great experiences with all of the social workers. You would totally love them because they are all exactly like you. It is sooooo sickening. I didn't realize there were more of you out there (ha, ha). We talked in depth about my anxiety and OCD and it was a relief to hear that, when she worked for the county, she always considered it a strength/asset when somebody sought help and continued receiving therapy and medication.

Even though the adoption process has been surprisingly enjoyable, I think the emotional aspect of it really hit me hard after our interview yesterday. At the end of the interview, we scheduled out the rest of our meetings, including the final home walk through and the time required for Katie to write the actual home study, and we figured out we will probably be certified and considered a "family available" by the end of October or early November. I think that realization broke down a wall I still had up surrounding my desire to have more children. I knew how strong the desire was, but I don't think I have ever really felt it before last night. For various reasons, I have never allowed myself to want more children. After so much time and so many losses, at some point I began to believe there was a reason why Jack and I were not able to have any more children. I still sometimes feel like we are not worthy or capable. Maybe it's my OCD, but it feels as though, if I acknowledge the incredible emotional response I have at the thought of finally having another child/children to raise, then it will all fall apart. My "what ifs" kick in: what if Jack and I should not really stay together, what if we fight, what if you and Dr. Weiss don't really think it's a good idea to adopt, what if we don't pass the home study, what if it causes problems with Grant, what if my anxiety and OCD come back. Well, my response to all of that is FORGET the *what ifs* and FORGET OCD! I am super happy and super excited to be on this journey.

I'm not sure if I've mentioned this, but I am on Step Seven in my daily devotional and workbook and have spent a few weeks exploring how God restores the crushed spirit of the humble if we come to Him with our defects in character, as we recognize we are incapable of controlling our unmanageable lives, and ask Him to remove our shortcomings. Well, in the previous steps, I have uncovered many, but I'm sure not all, of my defects and have found my worst ones tend to be pride and fear (avoidance). I have asked God to remove them, but as we all know, He sometimes works very slowly. I have also learned that part of Step Seven is I become willing to move out of my own way and act differently than I normally would in the moment. Normally, in a moment like this, I would not express how I am feeling nor would I acknowledge I might need anyone to help me through this process. As we both know, my fear and OCD would keep me from speaking and my pride would most certainly keep me from asking for support. In the last few weeks, I have realized what an important part of my life both you and the women's group have become for me. Ha, ha you have all become pieces of my puzzle. Find *those* pieces under your couch. That is super messed up for you guys! However, it is great for me because you have provided me with so many opportunities to act differently in the moment and begin to allow God to do His work.

I read "Letter to my Future Son" in my women's group this evening. I cried for the first time in group. I was like Niagara Falls. I needed this night—even if the adoption doesn't happen—because I am allowed to be hopeful that we will soon be able to add a son to our family. Tomorrow we have our individual interviews with Katie and our final home walk through will be the week after that. I am happy and can't wait to see who God has been preparing us to adopt. Dr. Weiss, my psychiatrist, suggested that this letter could also be representative of my more mature self who is speaking to my damaged/child self in addition to the child I foresee being placed with our family.

Letter to My Future Son

We have never met, but there is a place in my heart that has been prepared just for you. There is no one in this world who fits into it as perfectly as you—jagged edges and all. My hope for you, and for me, is for the Lord to guide me with His loving hands so I might have the courage and the patience and the strength to fill in the broken parts of your heart and your mind and your soul with love, kindness, and gentleness. The kind of love only a mother can provide. I know you have been through terrible times and, even though it was sometimes scary or painful or confusing, I know that the place you came from will always hold a special place in your heart. If you ever ask, I will always be willing to share that place with you because it has shaped who you are and has changed who I am.

The Lord has poured out His blessings upon our family in overflowing abundance so that we might be able to pour them out onto you. We have much to offer you: you will always have a warm, safe place to call home; you will never be hungry; your clothes will always fit; you will always be clean; you will be given the best education available; you will be given the opportunity and the resources to explore any interest or talent you have; you will be read to every night until you are able to read every night to us; you will have an amazing big brother who has been praying for you long before I ever thought to; you will have an equally amazing Nana who is waiting to smother you with love; and you will have a mom and a dad who will eternally and unconditionally love, protect, and guide you.

Those blessings are all needed and wonderful, but I think the greatest gift I have to share with you is my pain—my brokenness—my invisible scars. I want you to know where I have been so you will not feel like you need to hide from your truth or suffocate from the weight of your pain. I, too, have cried to the Lord, "Why?" only to be met with silence. The Lord has allowed me to feel the sting of betrayal and abandonment by people who were supposed to love and protect me. The Lord has allowed me to feel the loneliness and despair of anxiety and depression that led me down the path of drug abuse. The Lord has allowed me to feel the loss of hope in the depths of suicidal thoughts. Despite how difficult those times were for me, it has been in them where I learned some of my most important life lessons: I learned how to have mercy and forgiveness; I learned patience and surrender; I learned that the Lord will descend all the way to hell to rescue me if I call on Him.

A part of me believes the Lord allows us to suffer because only those who have truly experienced hell will be able recognize heaven when they see it.

You are my son now, and even though I have never seen your face, I know there is a glimpse of heaven in it. You will always be my child through all the good and all the bad this life has to offer. We will face it together in all our brokenness. You will never be alone again.

Love always,
Mom

This is a special journal for me. Until this point, I really could not remember much regarding my childhood, but recently I have been able to picture it more clearly. Yesterday Rachael and I talked about whether or not my childhood had really been as nice as I remembered. This journal is the result of that conversation. I feel like my lack of willingness to discuss my family/childhood has left a gaping hole in my recovery. This journal has been one of the more difficult ones for me to write because I knew I planned on sharing it. It marks the return of my ability to produce a coherent life story. I can fully remember—the gaps and fragments are gone.

Childhood Memories

Over the last couple of years, I have really questioned if the uneventful, yet pretty good, childhood I remembered, had actually occurred or if I had lived an altogether different life than my sketchy memory would allow. I mean, really, people like me and my sister simply are not produced by uneventful, yet pretty good, childhoods (or maybe that is some rule I invented). At the start of my recovery journey I only had a vague recollection of how I felt and my experiences as a child. I believe, and still do to an extent, that I had a childhood many people would kill to have because it was filled with married/loving parents, music lessons, good schools, and family vacations, yet everything I could remember was very general. I knew I had been a stubborn, yet fearful, child and I had also been a happy, yet introverted, child; however, I could not find within my internal filing system any substantive or real examples of why or how I became all of those things. Those memories have not returned in the flash flood I imagined, but in a slow, warm trickle of thoughts flowing in and flowing out of my mind. Yes, the childhood I had remembered did exist, yet so did a childhood I could not express or understand because, as a child, I did not have the awareness or capacity to see or know what was happening. I think it is also difficult to describe because there was no single event or tragedy that brought numbness to my life, but there was an underlying panic and fear buzzing beneath the surface year after year after year.

My dad was awesome and I was always very proud of the fact that he was a sergeant with the LAPD. He was a real life badass shooting bank robbers, saving babies and all sorts of stuff like that, but he was also a very loving and involved father. My dad was the one who taught me how to read. We would sit at a table in my bedroom and I would read *Little Bear* to him. I would get furious when I couldn't sound out a word and he wouldn't tell me what it was. I would scream and cry and pound the table—a combination of severe stubbornness and a severe need to get it right—to know the answer. My dad showed incredible patience and humor during those times and always came back to read again with me. My dad taught me how to ride a bike, change the oil and tire on a car, and how to drive. He also drove me to shelter after shelter to find the perfect cat, and he totally caved when we found two perfect kittens to bring home. My dad was the one who drove the long drive to St. Mary's Hospital when I was seventeen knowing they would be admitting me that evening for substance abuse. I don't remember exactly what we talked about, but I do remember he was loving and supportive and knew I needed help. I think, if I had to answer the question of who comforted me as a child, I would have to say it was my dad. Unfortunately, he was very rarely home due to working countless hours of overtime to support us.

My mom was a good mom and she did her best to take care of my sister and me. My mom would make special days for me when my sister was in school and would tell me how important it was to her to have individual time with each of us. We would walk down to the bakery and I would always get the same thing: a cinnamon crisp. It was always one of my favorite memories. My mom has always covered for me and has done everything she could to protect me in tough situations. She covered for me when I was sixteen and had begun getting into trouble by hanging out with the kind of people who break the law and use drugs. She covered for me when she found out I was sexually active (since she knew my dad would shoot anybody who came near me), and she made sure I had the knowledge and the means to be safe. My mom was there for me when Grant was born and I returned home with a 10 pound baby and a difficult C-section. She was there for me when I separated from Jack, and she had the self-control and the foresight to not say anything she would regret if we got back together. I have always appreciated that. So, I guess, if I had to answer the question of who has comforted me the most as an adult, I would have to say my mom. Unfortunately, I rarely see her due to the fact that I have not made my relationship with her a priority over the last several years.

That is the childhood I remember in concrete detail and nameable emotions. The childhood I do not remember is much more abstract, but it is the one that has caused me to seek escape. My only real understanding comes retrospectively from conversations I have had as an adult with other people. My parents did the best they could despite their ridiculously awful upbringings. My dad was born in Germany to a single mother right in the middle of WWII where he was bombed, moved from caregiver to caregiver, abused, and lived with his mother in a hospital for a year. Upon immigrating to the US when my dad was ten, my grandmother married a man who was very abusive. Due to his language barrier, my dad also struggled in school, so he decided to join the police force thinking it was his only option. Probably not a great idea for someone who had already been pretty traumatized, but he enjoyed the intensity of the job. Over time he felt very trapped and smothered by his job and became progressively more burnt out on his job and on Los Angeles. In 1984 my dad worked 30 twelve hour shifts in a row because the Olympics were in LA that year. Sometime shortly after, he had what has been referred to simply as a nervous breakdown. I remember finding him several times when I had gotten up in the middle of the night just sitting in the chair in the living room staring into space. Over the years I became much more aware of his anxiety and tension especially in the chaos created by my sister who, as it turns out, probably had undiagnosed bipolar disorder. They had violent arguments I still don't fully understand. My dad's behavior never really struck me as odd or abnormal. It was just the way he was, and it was something with which I could identify. He always told me he had tried to get help for his anxiety, but nothing had worked. Maybe that is where I got that rule.

My mom also experienced severe abuse and neglect as a child. Her parents each had three children when they married and had her, so both her parents and siblings were considerably older. Her father was an alcoholic who sexually abused her and her mother was bipolar and left her in her crib for long lengths of time. My mom's older siblings have told her they were not allowed to play with her or buy her things and she was treated horribly as a child. Considering this childhood background and the fact that my dad was often absent both in body and mind, I think my mom did a miraculous job caring for us. However, I think she suffered from severe depression and anxiety. When I was a young adult, she told me she had considered suicide when my sister and I were very young. As a child I would often find her crying but would never know why. She would be unpredictable in her moods. I have always thought she was dying. She would go into her room and cry saying she had chest pain or a migraine. I would sit outside her door not sure what to do. I always thought she was having a heart attack or a brain aneurysm. I felt very inadequate, very helpless, and very scared.

Making sense in that world is pretty much impossible: two awesome and loving parents consumed by mental illness. Hmmmm, that sounds a little familiar. Hoping to break that cycle!

Hopeless Moments

It is not so much that I want to die. It is that living has become too hard. I do not think there can be a deeper, darker thought than that of death. What a vicious monster I have found. I should have turned away, but I couldn't and now it's too late. I looked and now it's looking back. We are locked eye to eye and fist to fist as we fall swiftly, deeper and deeper into the abyss. A branch, a twig, a ledge, a rock—sometimes they slow the fall, but there is no denying the place at the end of it all. Into the chasm of my mind I fall as I battle the demon that is death and his seductive, evil call. I want to disappear.

I am a fake. Everything has always appeared good, but I have always hidden my core which I have always known was rotten and hollow. Anxiety—I hate it! It hijacks my mind and my body. I feel as though I cannot breathe. As though I will never breathe again—and I want it to stop—NOW. I am being tortured by the strangling grip of my life. The world is ultimately a terrible place to be—filled with evil and sadness and sin and suffering. I want to leave.

Satan sold an apple to a couple who already owned all the orchards in the world. Now he has tempted me. He has promised me everything. He has promised me air while I am suffocating. He has promised to make it all go away. Satan lays a thin, translucent layer over God's beautiful creation. I walk through Paradise, but it is hidden. I cannot distinguish between God's Eden and the devil's earth and I am no longer willing to try. I can no longer fight for a God who has abandoned me. Deep in my thoughts is where Satan dwells—the screams—the shouts of his living hell. No matter which direction I turn, the fire gets hotter as I slowly burn. Twisting, fighting, struggling more—I am simply unable to find the door. I am tired of looking.

My wandering soul is weary and tired. I no longer stand at an intersection of life—but on the edge of despair. I find myself once again alone—staring deeply into the abyss. I have wandered far from home...far from God and my heart beats faintly and searches aimlessly. God cannot be found at the bottom of the abyss. I have fallen too far.

I finished Step Eight which has been, by far, my personal favorite. I wrote out a bunch of boring shit like lists of people I had harmed, but I like this better. There is much more feeling to it—if you know what I mean. It's a little abstract, but essentially breaks down into three parts/areas of destruction in which I have caused harm: harm to myself, harm to innocent people in my life, and harm to my relationship with my husband and with God.

Willing to Make Amends
(Step 8)

The destruction lies not only in the chaos of my madness
But in the quiet calm found in the depths of suicidal sadness
Hanging here in tattered shreds are the pieces of my heart
Thrown like stones into the water—causing stillness to depart
I failed to guard it above all things—not seeing the ripple effect
Bringing silence to its life song rhythm—no beat can I detect
Is there a way to bring it back to life once more?
A way to help find peace in a bloody, civil war?

The destruction lies not only in my raging, screaming voice
But in the breaths that follow from a heart that's made a choice
My finely sharpened words cutting neatly into threads
Innocent lives turned upside down and on their tiny, little heads
Dishes of anger and of hate served to the guiltless undeserving
Knowing the food was quickly eaten is really quite unnerving
Can the damage be repaired by such a wretched, worthless soul?
Is there a way to once again make these blameless people whole?

The destruction lies not only in my trembling hands of human vice
But in the streams of poison flowing through my veins of ice
Two slowly shattered spirits traveling down this winding road
Have led each one the other to a place that does erode
The soul, the mind, the heart of any living, breathing being
The Lord cries out in sorrow at the tragedy He's seeing
Is there a way to repair the loving bond that has been torn?

Yes, says the Lord—when out of two, one is born

And the two are united into one. Since they are no longer two but one, let no one split apart what God has joined together—Mark 10:8-9

Christmas Cantata

Christmas Cantata at church tonight! Two years ago, I was high at the Cantata. High on weed and high on anxiety. I was dying. I was really dying. Mostly from hopelessness—but also from desperation. One year ago, at the Cantata—as my beautiful boy sang—as my beautiful boy caught a glimpse of me out of the corner of his eye—I realized he was searching for me. It planted a permanent reason to live in my mind and in my heart. This year at the Cantata—On This Very Night—I sat in peace in the presence of the Holy Spirit as He poured out His glorious light. I <u>know</u> there is joyous music and singing and dancing and light in heaven. Lord—I pray for continued peace in the hearts of me and my family. Thank you for your love! Amen!

III.

In God's Hands

Year Three: 2016

The Escape Artist

I am an escape artist—as all addicts are in some form or another. It is always about breaking free—of a situation, of an event, of a person, of an emotion, of a memory, of a possibility, of a loss, of an unattainable desire. I could go on for quite some time with the list, but the bottom line is that an addiction is always, always, always about how to "Get the hell out of Dodge!"

For the most part I have always been able to escape inward—which often allows my destructive behavior/addiction to go unnoticed for considerable amounts of time. As a child I always found comfort by escaping into my mind. This was mainly done through reading which, of course, was highly praised. This was also when I began to have what I can now identify as OCD thoughts and behaviors. Concealed within my mind those things helped me escape my anxiety and fears. My lifelong addiction to obsessive thoughts and compulsive behaviors had begun.

As I grew older, I sought other ways to escape. I was never pressured into smoking, drinking, or using drugs. I sought out the people and situations in which I knew I could find those things. I loved the way they made me feel. I no longer felt uncomfortable around people. I was around people who were not judgmental or critical. I was accepted by them—but most of all—my mind faded— my thoughts faded—I felt like I had truly escaped the heavy weight of my life.

There are many ways to escape the world and true addicts know the most effective methods. Sex, gambling, drugs, porn, video games, cutting, OCD, and eating disorders instantly remove a person from a swirling reality. Even if it is just for a moment—it feels worth the relief. It feels worth the risk.

I think there is a misconception in the world that hope resides in all the happy, crappy moments of our lives. That is bullshit. True hope can only exist in moments when all seems lost. The greatest hope can only exist in the most unlikely of places.

Finding Hope

Hope is not found on the mountain top where snowflakes fall and angels call. It sits in the fiery pits of hell where the devil dances when the music stops and thirsty souls drink from dry, empty wells.

Hope is not found in the joyous spring flower where sun drops gleam and angels scheme. It grows in fall's scattered seeds where the devil laughs at his ever-growing power and sinful souls whither like the leaves.

Hope is not found in the newborn's cry where rivers flow and angels tiptoe. It swims in the tears of the forsaken when the devil whispers, "I love you, now die," and lonely souls search for dreams that were taken.

Hope is not found in the newlyweds' kisses where eyes grow narrow and angels aim with cupid's arrow. It hides in the dark holes of the heart where the devil brags of thoughts so vile and dirty souls wash with filthy rags.

Hope is not found in the raised fist of the champion where anthems play and angels sway. It hangs upon the fingertips of those about to fall as the devil pries each finger one by one and heavy souls cry helpless calls.

In places where it is no longer needed hope does not reside, but it sits with the Lord in dark corners of the world as the lost souls confide. In order to find hope it must first be lost, where heaven and hell intersect, and the Lord touches earth and then pulls back. The light is best seen in the black.

Small Group Discussion

One of the really awesome things about being a Christian is that we are called to help carry each other's burdens and encourage one another. We are also called to hold up and support people when they are unable to stand on their own. I am blessed to be part of a small group consisting of people who believe in and live out these commands. I have already mentioned some of my struggles to the group over various times, so they were at least generally aware that I have struggled with severe anxiety and depression over my life, but they did not know about the extent of my OCD or what it really meant. There are also a couple of people, Rick and Becky, who know most of the fine details of my struggles. The group is also very much involved and a part of our family's adoption journey and I am grateful to have them in my life.

I decided after texting you that I was going to bring up how much I was struggling with the return of my anxiety and OCD recently and the effects they have on my faith. I went into detail about how OCD is all about control and doubt and how the unknowns of adopting had, in large part, triggered the worsening of my symptoms. I explained how OCD tells me I have control of things such as whether we get a placement, whether it will be successful, and the number of children we will get. I did not tell them how my mind believes the number of Christmas stockings I hang up or the way I close my car door gives me the power to control these unknowns, or if I don't do certain things, then it will cause a negative outcome. I told them about the fear of losing my sanity, but I did not tell them about the sexual or violent harming intrusive thoughts. I told them I can accept whomever God wants to send to us (one or two, ages, circumstances, challenges, even the timing), but it is in the waiting where I fall apart because it is in the waiting where I have the opportunity to go insane. It is not that I have to have a child immediately. It is the fear that my unknown/undiscovered insanity or my unknown/uncontrollable harming and sexual impulses will be revealed before we are able to adopt—even though, of course, these thoughts are horrific and disturbing to me. It is like half of my mind stands helplessly and hopelessly by as it watches the other half slip into oblivion.

I also told the group how much I valued the fact that I could tell them these things about myself and rely on them for support. I even cried. It was totally badass!! The responses from the group varied, but they were all positive and helpful in their own way. Most of the women in the group have struggled with some sort of mother-related issues (miscarriage, infertility, post-partum depression) and many of the people have worked through depression and anxiety related issues. Funny—none of them thought I was crazy or unfit to be a parent—even after I told them how crazy I was. Not one of them questioned my faith. Rick told me the thoughts are not me and that Jack and I are two of the best people he has ever known (and he's pretty old). Claudine offered to round up anything I put on a list in case we are surprised or unable to prepare before the placement—she is also the one who will be there to remind me I am not crazy. Becky is always a phone call or cup of coffee away if I need to talk. When we prayed—it was the women who knew what I needed most. Like I said recently, I have an amazing network of resources to rely on when we finally do get a placement. All of this was awesome, but I think the best part of talking with the group was how it affected Jack. After we got home, he told me how great it was that I had shared with the group. He also seemed to understand better why the wait is so hard for me. Now that is some good stuff!!!

Not to be dramatic, but living with OCD is a little like living in every horror movie ever created; however, it is mostly like living in the seventh or eighth sequel of *A Nightmare on Elm Street* with its ridiculously implausible situations, yet equally terrifying realization that, no matter which weapons or tactics are used, this monster is going to just keep coming back to terrorize and destroy the lives of innocent people. Rather than the temporary suspension of disbelief required to enjoy such films, OCD is more of a permanent suspension of disbelief in which the most absurd thoughts and ideas are perceived as true or possible. I have already described my sexual

OCD regarding animals, children, and homosexuality, so I have decided I should add a little insight into some other areas.

My first OCD thoughts revolved around the fear of being contaminated by household products. My mom had used some powdery Comet cleanser in the shower and warned me not to touch it because it was poisonous. I think I was around six or seven. After that, every time I took a shower, I believed that the cleanser came up through the drain and would most likely kill me. I tried not to breathe the steam. I tried not to step on the drain. I tried to wash the invisible enemy off of my feet so my feet would not accidentally contaminate the rest of my body. When I was a child, I thought the vapor from the frying pans and the aerosols from deodorant or hair spray would cause me to develop Alzheimer's, so I began holding my breath until the tiny monsters were gone. Hmmm, maybe that was around the time I forgot how to breathe.

OCD causes me to doubt my sanity and my ability to stay connected to the world—when I was a teenager, I was certain I was developing schizophrenia. I checked and rechecked my mind and my ability to think. This is also when I began to fear that a lack of or inability to sleep would cause me to go crazy and I would be taken away from everything I knew and placed in an institution. Also as a teenager, I always thought I was dying from cancer or HIV. I believed I could smell cancer on my hands and clothes and changed and washed until I could no longer smell it. Sometimes I could not get rid of the smell. I also believed I had contracted HIV by swimming in a pool with a girl who told me a bully had started a rumor that she had AIDS even though she didn't. I began spending many hours researching the signs, symptoms, and contractibility of many different, but always life threatening and incurable, health problems. Keep in mind this was in the 1980's and early 90's, before the Internet, and required a large amount of effort. I constantly checked to see if I was developing symptoms and constantly calculated the statistical chances of developing these diseases.

Contamination and death and dying obsessions have remained throughout my entire life. At one point, I could not touch anything green because I would be ingesting rat poison. If I bumped against something or found a scratch, it meant I was going to develop tetanus. I would always check to see how deep a wound was and check to see if the object could have given me tetanus. I thought I was going to get rabies because a dog drooled on my shoe, or because Samson ate a dead animal that had probably been chewed on by a rabid skunk or raccoon, or because I was bitten by a duck (because, even though birds don't get rabies, some sort of animal with rabies must have come into contact with it causing it to carry the virus), or by touching a walnut shell that most definitely was eaten by a rabid squirrel. I thought I was going to get HIV from the needles I used as a dialysis tech. I replayed withdrawing the needles to make sure I hadn't stuck myself without realizing it. I checked my hands for little red dots to make sure I hadn't been stuck. I was convinced that any type of red mark was a sign I had been stuck with a contaminated needle. I also thought I would get HIV by sharing a desk with someone who had HIV and by using the same door or the same phone or the same stapler. I think the HIV thing, and maybe even the homosexuality stuff, stem from my upbringing. My parents both always spoke very negatively about homosexuals and considered them to be disgusting, disturbed, sick, etc. My dad would always point out when he thought he saw a gay couple and I could never figure out how he knew. He would say things like two men sitting together in a movie meant they were gay or a woman with short hair meant she was a lesbian. He also very much connected HIV to homosexuality. He told me HIV was God's way of getting rid of bad groups of people (drug addicts and homosexuals). That is completely messed up thinking!!!! I do not feel that way, but that is what I was taught by my parents.

The harming OCD came after Grant was born in 2003. I have already given some details on this, but the main idea is I was concerned I would be unable to control myself and impulsively hurt him or I would hurt him without realizing it (this might be connected to the fear of going crazy and not being able to stay connected to reality) or that he would simply, suddenly not exist anymore as if he had been a figment of my imagination. My OCD made me think tapping ten times in a row in sets of four would prevent these things from happening. My OCD kept me in his room every night for countless minutes and hours so I could pet his head the right way and the right number of times. Any sharp objects had to be stored out of sight. Knives could not be placed together in the dishwasher and had to be placed sharp side down. I had to take four sips of anything I drank, and if I didn't sip the exact same amount each time, I had to start over. God, this shit is making me tired!!!!

I still occasionally have the harming OCD, but I think I am currently struggling mostly with the fear of losing my mind or doing something impulsive. My OCD tells me if I am not asleep by a certain time, then I will never fall asleep, causing me to go crazy and either be institutionalized or die. If I do not lay a certain way or wear a certain shirt or take a certain number of breaths, then I will become sick causing me to be unable to sleep, causing me to go crazy. OCD causes me to think what I accept as reality and truth is an illusion of a delusional mind. Children cannot just disappear out of thin air— that is, unless they never existed to begin with. OCD tells me I will lose my mind through schizophrenia, Alzheimer's, rabies, lead poisoning, or even lack of sleep. OCD causes me to doubt my safety—it tells me I will lose my life through HIV, tetanus, asbestosis, cancer, and contamination/poisoning by household substances. OCD swallows me alive. I even think my suicidal thoughts have shifted into the realm of OCD. I know (at least I think I know), I do not currently want to kill myself (I just don't say it because I am afraid I am tricking myself and the people around me). My suicidal thoughts consist of checking the statistics and checking the lists to see how "suicidal" I really am. I also have thoughts that I will impulsively kill myself or will at some point not be able to stop myself even though I do not want to commit suicide. The night a couple of weeks ago when I told group about my suicidal thoughts, the thoughts had occurred while I was drying my hair. I was standing next to a large tub of water (for the turtle tank) and was overcome with the thought that I would not be able to prevent myself from standing in the water and dropping the hair dryer. This is the type of thing I have lived with for as long as I can remember. Different obsessions—same OCD. It is my real life (and don't tell me it's not real) Freddy Krueger.

The Call

Desiree, our social worker from Lilliput, called today. It was the call we have been waiting for since beginning the adoption process a year ago. We are going to a disclosure meeting for two brothers—Isaiah and DeAngelo—ages eight and five. We had originally told Desiree we did not want a child under the age of five, but Jack, Grant and I all feel that the ages of these boys are a more natural fit for our family.

We are super excited! I am nervous, but I have a good feeling about the meeting.

Lord—please clear the path needed for us to complete our family. Thank you for carrying us this far. I know we are safe in Your arms.

—Amen

Yes!

Yesterday's disclosure meeting was amazing. We learned so much about Isaiah and DeAngelo. We said YES to bringing the boys into our family today. Desiree handed us over to our new social worker, Marie. We are so excited and so grateful for the love in our lives.

These boys are not loved because they are perfect or beautiful, but they are perfect and beautiful because they are loved. I have never met them, but they are my beloved boys. Thank you, Lord, for allowing me to feel and express unconditional love.

—Amen

Trust the Lord with all your heart and lean not on your own understanding. Seek His will in all your ways and He will make straight your paths—Psalm 3:5-6

DeAngelo

Origin: African-American, Greek, Latin
Meaning: From the angel/messenger of God

The world falls back together—in pieces—one by one
The path becoming clear in the image of a son
Held tightly in the arms of love—the hands of his Creator
Sent to mend a shattered heart and heal a sinful hater
Not the story I had written in my broken, battered mind
Something better—something bigger—has been left for me to find
A life—a breath—taken by the Lord—then exhaled eternally
We are but visitors passing through—together—him and me
Looking towards the promise of a new story—a new beginning
Time stands still for just a moment—then the world continues spinning

The skies open up their gates—releasing angels—one by one
Delivering God's messenger as a beautiful, begotten son

Gliding gently towards the bonds of earth and climbing from the pits of hell, a glimpse of paradise peeks through his eyes with stories he longs to tell

Joy flowing from the heart pierced by unconditional, undying love
Is the star hope makes its wishes on as it gazes at heaven above

In the deepest, darkest places—God places hope throughout the land, and in my pain, I see a child smiling brightly as joy reaches out its hand

A faith, a hope, a love discovered as our lives have been made new
I am reminded as God whispers to me always—**I can't stop loving you**

What If This Works?

I am exhausted. This is a really difficult journey and sometimes I just get tired. I want the boys here tomorrow, but I need to be patient and allow for the transition process. Rather than focusing on "what if this fails," I need to focus on "what if this works"—because focusing on the negative will not cause it to hurt less if a loss occurs.

If this works:

- I will have three beautiful boys whom the Lord has entrusted me with to guide and love
- I will have a house filled with laughter and love
- Grant will be a big brother
- All of my struggles would have led me to this joy
- St. Joseph's will gain two new students
- Isaiah and DeAngelo will have the family they need and deserve
- I will have challenges I could never have predicted
- I will have the experience of surrendering and trusting God to take care of the details of my life
- All of the bedrooms will be full
- Heaven will gain two new souls
- Two new souls will gain heaven

--Amen!

The Lord has spoken! Isaiah and DeAngelo are in our family. They moved in today. What an enormous and unexpected blessing they have been in the short time we have known them. I love them and will follow the path God has chosen for us. Lord, guide us and keep us close as we follow and seek Your will. Thank you for loving me.

--Amen

I Will Hold Your Hand

I will hold your hand until the day I die—I will hold your hand. Your tiny fingers have wrapped themselves around my heart and now I can't let go. Your laughter fills my dreams as it dances wildly and free. Your tears drain my heart as they trickle one by one and sometimes all at once. I will hold your hand until the day I die—I will hold your hand. I will send you off to fly above your highest dreams, but I will always have your hand in mine to show you the way back home. When I am gone, I will wait for you at heaven's edge to hold your hand again and I will be holding the flower you gave me.

Sometimes things happen that can make a person truly realize how deeply connected we are.

My soul changed its shape the day I met you. It will never return to the way it was—and it would never want to. You make it shine— even when my heart aches—my soul remembers you. There is nothing more beautiful than unconditional love. The only thing more beautiful than feeling unconditional love is watching how it affects the heart and the soul of the one who is being unconditionally loved. The Lord has allowed me to experience this—there is no greater gift that can be given. It is worth the pain and the fear of losing it.

Letter to My Children

I want you to know what I have done so I could be with you today.

I have chosen to walk in the sun's revealing light over hiding in the safety of the shadow's cover of darkness as the sun beat mercilessly down on my exposed heart, mind, and soul threatening to burn out the essence of each as it revealed my thoughts, my weaknesses, and my doubts.

I did this so you will know there is no sin too great to be overcome by the grace of God.

I have stared deeply into the eyes in the mirror as they vowed to take the last breath of life from my body and as they spoke of hopelessness and contempt for this world, and I have forgiven them for their lack of understanding and their lack of love for me—and for you.

I did this so you will know the battle raging within you can and will be won if you are willing to surrender.

I have allowed myself to thirst and to starve as I searched this world for a God I had been hiding from all of my life—only to find Him sewing the pieces of my heart back together as He wept for His lost and lonely child.

I did this so you might have the opportunity to drink from the rivers of living water and eat of the bread of life that gives eternal hope to those who hunger for it.

I have climbed mountain tops where I placed letters to the Lord in mailboxes that touched the heavens, and I have traveled rivers, peaceful yet untamed, that have carried me to heaven's edge where I have seen a glimpse of the glory of God, and I have turned around, at His command, to come down from the peak, and I have gotten back into the boat without hesitating.

I did this so I could come back for you, and I would do it again tomorrow so I could be with you today.

Jesus said to them, 'I am the bread of life; whoever comes to me shall not hunger, and whoever believes in me shall never thirst—John 6:35-36

Love,
Mom

One Step Closer

The judge terminated reunification services for the boys' birthmother today. I cannot imagine the grief she is experiencing as she realizes her hope of getting back her children is not going to happen. The next step will be terminating her parental rights.

I think God has planned for these boys to stay in our lives. Either way—they are our sons forever. I love them more than I ever dreamed I would. The Lord has been preparing my heart for this moment this whole time. I am scared of not being capable or adequate enough for Isaiah and DeAngelo, but that is because I have forgotten who has placed me on this path.

I need to trust in the Lord's plan.

Pastor Smith-

It has been a long time since we have spoken, and I have realized in that time what an important piece of my recovery you are. In the year since our second youth conference in Colorado, I have recalled, many times, the beauty of watching the Lord's hand reach down from heaven to release the pain and the shame that had been locked up in the hearts of our youth. Being able to share my life with you and the youth there was a gift from God, and I often find my mind escaping to that glimpse of paradise. Much has changed since then. I'm sure you could have predicted, and I think you even cautioned me, that my life would be filled with an onslaught of spiritual warfare upon my return to the valley. That was an accurate prophesy!

In many ways since then the Lord has blessed me beyond measure with His glorious plans for me. The most beautiful blessing being the two boys, Isaiah and DeAngelo, He has placed into our hearts and home. The boys are five and eight and have been with us for a few months. The biological mother's parental rights will be terminated in August and they will be free for adoption. The boys have been welcomed into the loving hands of God and the Body of Christ that is the church. I have watched in awe as they have received the Holy Spirit in their lives manifested in the experience of unconditional love and miraculous healing of the heart. They are truly the most beautiful people I have ever seen, and their presence transcends anything I might have planned for my life. They have a long way to go, but I am certain they are exactly where the Lord intends for them to be.

So, why then, with so much joy in my life, have I fallen back into anxiety, depression, OCD, and even suicidal thoughts (don't worry...I am receiving professional help)? Watching the tragedy of these boys losing their mother and a mother losing her children has been too painful for me to watch. I have closed my eyes and fallen asleep to God's will in my life. Satan knows my weaknesses and has preyed mercilessly upon them. He reminds me of how the Lord has prevented me from having more children because I cannot be trusted with much. Satan reminds me that this dream I am having will soon be over, and I will once again awaken to the nightmare of what I really deserve. Satan reminds me that part of me wants to leave this world a little early, and he has laid many plans before me, and I have played each one through in my head. Thankfully, God has placed a flaw in each one of the evil one's plans and promises causing none to be suitable for me.

I am reaching out to you for prayer and spiritual guidance. My faith has once again been crushed and I am unable to feel hope in this world.

Thanks,
Michelle

Rachael-

Pastor Smith and I talked for close to an hour on Tuesday. I had planned on talking about faith and prayer and stuff like that, but we surprisingly spoke very little on the topics. Other than a prayer at the beginning and two biblical references at the end, there was no mention of the spiritual. I suppose he felt it was better to keep things purely at the level in which we are currently stuck. You know that icky, complicated human level where emotions love to play. We spoke mainly of love and fear and grief—my three favorite topics! NOT!! Pastor Smith's sons were six and eight when they joined his family through adoption, so in addition to his pastoral training, he could relate on a very personal level. Simply put, we came to the conclusion that my current spiral is related to unresolved grief over my miscarriages, but I'm sure you already knew that.

Early on in the conversation we started discussing my fear of losing the boys and how that was connected to my pregnancy losses. He seemed to think that the fact that the boys are essentially the age my biological children would have been has messed with my mind. The age coincidence is not something I had given much thought to, but I think it is very significant. It is like seeing how "things would have been" if I had been able to carry my pregnancies to term. It feels like God is saying, "Oh, just kidding about that only child part." This causes me a ton of internal struggle because I have tried so hard not to view these children as "replacements" of the children I had hoped for, but as the unique individuals whom God has placed in our lives. It is also a little like a reversal of one of my OCD themes. Rather than the boys being a figment of my imagination that could, at any moment, disappear, it is more like they have been here all along and I just failed to notice them.

We also talked about self-care—blah, blah, blah—that Jack and I are and are not doing. He thinks I need to start running more and asking for help more—you can shut up and stop laughing now! Another area we discussed was when I started to go into this particular downward spiral which, as you know, began after meeting the boys' birth mother. Pastor Smith thinks the sadness I have regarding my losses has been triggered by watching this woman losing her children. He thinks I am relating to her more than I am to any other person in my life right now. I think that is true, but I don't know what to do with that information.

He told me to print out this verse and put it somewhere I would see it every day like the visor in my car. I am not certain that the two of you have never spoken or perhaps could even be the same person.

So, do not fear, for I am with you; do not be dismayed, for I am your God. I will strengthen you and help you; I will uphold you with my righteous right hand—Isaiah 41:10

I have realized how unable I was to grieve the loss of my pregnancies—the loss of my hoped-for family. I can now see what I had lost as I watch DeAngelo and Isaiah become part of our family. Before this I would never have allowed myself to feel or understand how much I had really lost. Parts of me have been missing. Parts of me were lost in those lives that lasted only for the blink of an eye. New and unexpected parts are filling in many of the holes and healing many of the wounds. They are neither better than nor less than any other part of me. They are equal in their profound beauty.

Thank God

Thank God I didn't know what to cry for—but now I finally do
Thank God I didn't know who I was missing was such a bright and beautiful you

For I would not have survived

Thank God I didn't see who you were when you went missing
Thank God I didn't see this face I now am kissing

For I would not have survived

Thank God I never heard your laugh or the cries of your brother
Thank God I never heard the breaking of my heart each time I lost another

For I would not have survived

Thank God I didn't know you were real and not just a dream of mine
Thank God I didn't know how I would stumble across you in God's gracious, precious time

For I would not have survived

Love and Loss

It is OK to feel the grief. It is OK to feel the love. Hiding does not make it feel any better. The great love I have for these boys has exposed a great sorrow that has been festering. Rain and tears can fall onto a beating heart, but they cannot make it love any less.

Of course, I am tired. My heart has been flooded with the most beautiful love and the deepest sadness all at once with no keeper at the gates. I trust the Lord has an awesome plan for my life.

Hey Soul Stealer

Who am I that you should fight so desperately for my worthless, ragged soul? I have always only wanted peace! Who am I that God should hand me over so easily when He dropped me as a child down the deep and lonely hole where you sat waiting patiently for me? No matter—I have come to accept that there are often more questions than answers.

Perhaps it was just the way the shadows fell, but everything looked like a black hole to me. I didn't know where the gun was, but you told me it was pointed in my direction. I believed that in the course of all the previous events, it was clear that something was bound to happen. You told me life would rear its ugly head to me. You left me with nothing to lose but my apathy.

I believed you when you said that the dice are loaded and everybody rolls with their fingers crossed. Everybody thinks that the war is over. Everybody thinks the good guys lost. You told me the fight was fixed. You said that's how it goes and everybody knows. You told me the boat was leaking and that the captain lied. You told me everybody has a broken feeling like their father or their dog just died.

You saw my red heart and painted it jet black. No colors anymore, you wanted them all black. You told me that my flowers and my love were never to come back. I saw the people turn their heads and quickly look away, because like a newborn baby, love dying happens every day. I looked inside myself and saw my heart turned black. No more red door to my inner soul. You helped me fade away and not have to face the facts. It's hard to look at life when my whole world is black.

Goodbye darkness. You are my old friend, but I'll never talk with you again. Because a vision that was planted in my brain no longer belongs to the realm of silence. In all my dreams I walked alone and you told me that would never change. You told me people talk without saying anything. You told me people hear without understanding. You said the sounds of silence should not be disturbed.

You did not disappoint me and you have never let me down. You should not feel guilty and there is no judgement waiting for you. You saw the end before it all began. Yes, you saw I was blinded and you knew you would win. You took what was you thought was yours by eternal right. You took my soul out and left me in the cold, dark night. You know me too well. I've been addicted to you. I could not have survived without you in those difficult times, but the time has finally arrived when I do not need you. You are causing more harm than good.

I am sorry, but you must leave. It is time to retire. I can live without OCD, anxiety, drugs, and depression. I can face the tragedy because I know the triumph that comes out of it. I can face the sadness because I know the healing it brings. I can face a discouraging and hurtful world because I have felt the love that hides in the hearts of strangers. Thank you for all you have done for me. Goodbye.

Love always,
Michelle

Two Years

I made it to two years! We all have the stomach flu. I'm calling it the Stomach Tsunami of 2016. Tonight, Isaiah is crying because he wants to go home. Lord, help us, guide us and walk with us as we help these children to heal and feel your love and ours.

—Amen

The Lord has spoken once again! Today we put an offer in on a house. It was accepted this evening. I am finally escaping the darkness of this house. I have been trying to get out of the hallway of this house for a long time. I have tried to reach for the door—but I have always stumbled—and I see how obdurate this house is—it does not want to be changed. It wants to keep things exactly as they are. It has me and it does not want to let me go. The old ego I am shedding tries to cling as I pick it away piece by flaking piece. I am not a butterfly who was once an ugly caterpillar. I am not a phoenix rising from the ashes. I am a snake who has left on the old skin for too long. I have forgotten the beauty of the scales underneath. I have refused to grow out of fear of the ugliness and tediousness of shedding my old self—my old, obdurate self.

In the In Between

In the in between is where I always wander much too far
And in the in between is where this saddened struggler cries
Stuck in between the way things always were and the way things
always are

**Stuck in between the truthful moment and the never-ending
lies**

In the passageways of my heart I have stood for far too long
Standing-looking-waiting
Not able to choose a door for fear that I was wrong
Loving turned to hating
And in my dreams I heard the pounding, beating of its song
Singing, chanting, "No more waiting! You have stood there far too
long."

In the corridors of my head I have walked myself into a wall
Marching-smiling-faking
Not knowing left then left, then left would lead me home after all
Crying before waking
And in my dreams I heard the grinding of the gears as they began to
stall
Screeching, screaming, "No more sleeping! You have walked into a
wall."

In the hallways of my soul I have surrendered who I am
Losing-lying-dying
Not able to escape as each new door would slam
Not really even trying
And in my dreams I heard the winding river as it swam
Whistling, whispering, "No more staying! It is time you gave a
damn."

In the in between is where I have been lost
And in the in between is where this silent struggler screams
Stuck in the hallway of this world frozen by its bitter frost

Stuck in the nightmare in between the waking moment and my dreams

Letter to Self as a Child

Michelle-

Every time I hear a wind chime, I think of you: the visible and the invisible coming together to sing an exquisite, but subtle, song. I owe you an apology. I left you behind and forgot about you. I pretended you didn't exist. In my mind you and your stupid, little childhood had never happened. Well, I am sorry, but I am also in the business of making amends, and this is the best I can do for you. I have come back to get you, to heal you, and to make you, once again, part of who I am. I am here to shake you up a bit. I am here to tell you how things really are and how things will really be—because I know for a fact no one else in your life ever will. They will hide things from you. They will lie. They will cover up who they really are and who they think the rest of the world is. It is too hard for them to see reality because they long ago learned to stop looking at it. I have been thinking about you a lot lately and there are a few things I need to share with you.

Your family: They love you, but mom and dad have never really learned how to be parents, and even more importantly, neither of them has ever experienced the unconditional love of a mother or a father. On the outside, they know how to look and act correctly, but inside, they are lost and alone—not even able to rely on or be honest with each other. They live separate lives because they are unable to genuinely connect to others. They are doing their best which is a hell of a lot better than their parents did for them; however, I know that sometimes their best falls far short of what you need. I also want to reassure you that your mom is not dying. She has migraines—not brain aneurisms. She has anxiety attacks—not heart attacks. She doesn't know it, but she suffers from anxiety and depression. She is not dying! However, your dad is totally crazy. He never recovered from his childhood and he views the world as a relentlessly growling monster. He is unable to see how he can get better. You cannot fix him and there will be times when you need him and he just isn't there; however, there will be many times he will catch you when you fall.

You: You are not shy! You are just very sensitive to how people feel. This is both a curse and a blessing. You will have a great capacity for compassion—a gift that will be used boldly by the Lord; however, you will also have a profound coldness to protect yourself from a deeply fallen humanity—a sadness that will be preyed upon heavily by the devil. I know you often feel crushed by the responsibility you feel towards others. It is ok for you to hide for now. It is your only defense in your chaotically rigid world. You will stumble in your search for meaning, but I promise you will eventually find the delicate balance that allows you to flow freely along God's living waters. You will not need to hold your breath forever. I promise you that.

The most important thing to remember as you stand at the beginning of your journey is that God is always working in your life! I know you are beginning to lose faith in His existence, but that is only because He has never been anything more than an obligation to you and your family. You have never been told of His love. I don't want to spoil it for you, but I can tell you that God has some amazing plans for you. He can and will perform undeniable miracles for you. You will walk with some of the most beautiful people He has to offer. I promise you He will always provide exactly what you need.

Love-
Michelle

Hell is a State of Mind

"Hell is a state of mind - ye never said a truer word. And every state of mind, left to itself, every shutting up of the creature within the dungeon of its own mind - is, in the end, Hell. But Heaven is not a state of mind. Heaven is reality itself. All that is fully real is Heavenly. For all that can be shaken will be shaken and only the unshakeable remains."
— C.S. Lewis

Despite my constant relapse into anxiety and depression, I have a profound awareness of God's loving presence in my life. That is an impossible, but unshakably true, fact in my life. I have absolutely no doubt that, as I stumbled through three decades as an atheist, the Lord was actively preparing me for unthinkably glorious moments. Even as I turned away in hopelessness, He placed in my vast and vacant heart the whispering echoes of His love that gently and slowly and patiently always led me back to Him. Probable impossibilities weave through my story. In places where there were once walls, there are now, of course, doors that are not even locked. Around each moment and under each detail I look with awe and disbelief at an atheist gone rogue in search of God who has looked back to find each moment has been planned with love and care. For some reason it is both beautiful and heartbreaking. It was not supposed to be this way, but there was no other way it could be.

I became a parent the first time because it was what I was supposed to do. I became a parent the second time because it was what I had been prepared to do. The Lord gives us a great responsibility when he places the most vulnerable yet most easily loved people into our lives. He gives us glimpses of paradise when he places the honor of parenting upon us. It is the closest we can come to experiencing heaven's beauty. God is the ultimate example of perfect parenting. He is not a helicopter parent, but He does occasionally save us from ourselves. He knows what we need while we can only see what we desire. He allows us to fall and to hurt and to lose because there is no better teacher, no better consequence, than having to live with ourselves and take responsibility for who we are. We can really only begin to understand God's love for us when we experience the love we have for our children. We don't love them because they are perfect, and we don't stop loving them because they scream, "I hate you!" The Lord teaches us the meaning of unshakeable love through our children—that is, if we are willing to open our hearts.

I was born with a broken heart, passed down by my parents, who were incapable and unwilling to believe that love, heaven, and God were anything but conditional. My goal as a parent is to allow my children to experience unconditional love so they might see God at work in their lives. That is an uplifting and hopeful goal. I do, however, always find my home in sadness. Maybe I return to sadness when I realize how much the Lord has given me in spite of how little I deserve (this is not a self-esteem or self-worth thing. It is strictly in the biblical sense). Grace is God's undeserved mercy, love, and forgiveness. I have been given much of it. It is at the same time everything I will ever need, yet it never seems to be enough—and so, I will always struggle. The world ensures I always return to the hell I have created instead of to the heart my Lord has prepared. I have heaven in my heart and hell in my head. That is not the way it is supposed to be, but it is who I am, and it is how God chooses to use me.

Christmas 2016

This year is what a miracle looks like. It is the face of God staring back at me. It is the sound of Satan being crushed by Love. It is hope breathed into a lifeless body. I am grateful there are five stockings hanging over our fireplace. Nothing is impossible with God. I am pretty sure that, when the last day of my life arrives, I will look back and count 2016 as one of the best years of my life. Such odd numbers really rub my OCD the wrong way. Three children—a family of five. I turned 41. No rhyme or reason to the numbers other than their strangeness, but they are the magic numbers I never would have chosen. They are the winning Lotto combination, but I have gained more than any amount of money. I have gained the priceless gift of my children.

Jesus looked at them and said, "With man this is impossible, but with God all things are possible."—Matthew 19:26

IV.

Love Never Fails

Year Four: 2017

We have but a short time to live
Like a flower we blossom and then wither;
Like a shadow we flee and never stay.
In the midst of life we are in death
(Book of Common Prayer)

In 1994 I was working as a dialysis technician in San Diego, but I don't remember exactly what I was doing when I heard her speak those quiet words. "You look so sad," she said. Geraldine was not one of the most-liked patients in the unit and was known for her often sour attitude, but in that moment, she became a loving, caring human being. I think I was standing by a disposal bin, my hands rushing to discard the blood-filled tubes so I could prepare for the next group of dialysis patients. I smiled and shook my head saying, "No, I am just very tired." In an effort to convince her of my lack of sadness, I sat with her for a few minutes to carry on a nonchalant conversation. In a way she was right. It was as though she saw right through me to things I could not even see for myself. However, in a way, she was also very wrong. I was not simply sad. I was smothered by the despair of death. I had entered healthcare as a young, delusional idealist who believed medicine could, and would, heal the world. I left healthcare in 1999 with the knowledge that people are rarely healed, but more commonly broken, by the industry they trust so much. I left having seen the faces and hearing the regrets of those about to die. I became unable to look at patients without envisioning their younger selves and how their lives could have been different. That was when I decided to become a teacher.

When all is quiet around me and I gently close my eyes, I can still recall each of their names even though more than 20 years have passed. I have tried to forget them, but the Lord has not allowed that to happen.

Ron Roberts—my first stick. Due to his Parkinson's disease, I couldn't tell if he was afraid of me or if he was just joking around. His shaking served as a good distraction, and I placed the needles perfectly into his arm. He patted me on the arm and smiled. My confidence soared and I was asked to stay on at the unit where I had trained. I felt at ease behind the mask and the gloves and the white lab coat. Even the most difficult patients, and there were many, began not only allowing me, but requesting for me, to be their tech. Olivia, a loud and obnoxious woman who initially cussed me out for looking like a sixteen year old coming at her with a needle, grew to trust me and I became one of only two people she would allow anywhere near her.

Whitey—my first code—and the only code who ever lived to return to our unit. He asked us why we had brought him back. He had been happy to die. On the bright side, he had lost about 30 years of his memory and had the pleasure of falling in love with his wife all over again. I remember how efficiently we worked on him like machines. I also remember the looks of horror on the patients around us. It was as though they were watching their near futures. I tried to become cold, but it was just too real. I cared too much. I connected too much. My already heavy world began to crush me. Death in our society is degrading and I watched for years as it consumed people I had come to know and love. I tried to leave, but I was trapped by the contract I had signed agreeing to commit to two years of service for the training I had received. I could have left if I had the $2000 to break the contract, but that was a fortune to me at the time.

Rosa Diaz—another code—I was on break when the alarm sounded. She was my patient, so I jumped in to perform chest compressions. Her chest, weakened by previous heart surgeries, cracked with the first push, but I continued when I was told that was not unusual. I could feel and hear her ribs rubbing against her crushed sternum. The crash cart was quickly brought over and we were able to begin giving breaths with the ambu-bag. As the techs tilted her head back and opened her mouth I could see her tongue was still green from the lollipop I had given her earlier. As the paramedics removed her on a stretcher, the theme song from MASH was playing on one of the TV sets. Every time I hear that song it reminds me of that day:

Suicide is Painless (Theme Song to MASH)

Through early morning fog I see
visions of the things to be
the pains that are withheld for me
I realize and I can see...

that suicide is painless
it brings on many changes
and I can take or leave it if I please.
I try to find a way to make
all our little joys relate
without that ever-present hate
but now I know that it's too late, and...

The game of life is hard to play
I'm gonna lose it anyway
The losing card I'll someday lay
so this is all I have to say.

The sword of time will pierce our skins
It doesn't hurt when it begins
But as it works its way on in
The pain grows stronger...watch it grin

It seems silly, but the experience has haunted me since that day and the song's lyrics have become even more meaningful to me in the last few years.

Kenny. Kenny was the catalyst for a bout of OCD lasting nearly ten years. He was HIV positive due to IV drug use. He often complained of itching and constantly pulled at his needles while on dialysis. Of course, he eventually pulled out the needle that pumps the blood back into the patient's body. Not that it matters, but I was relatively new to the unit and was completely unaware of his HIV status. Blood flew from the needle like water from a hose that has been let go of too soon. I immediately turned off the machine and placed pressure onto his graph that was also shooting blood. It was then that I realized he had also pulled out his other needle—the one that pulls blood out of the body. I placed pressure on the other bleeding hole in his arm. That needle had been taped a little better, so it remained on his arm shortly below the hole it had created. My finger was no more than a quarter of an inch away from it. He looked hard into my eyes and simply said, "Careful." It was only later that I discovered why he had been so concerned. That was in 1995. I was certain I had stuck myself without realizing it and found proof everywhere I looked on my hands. Every scratch and every dot. Every time I touched something sharp. Every time I saw something sharp, (because, of course, I could cut myself without knowing it) I became infected. That lasted until well after Grant was born in 2003.

Mr. Thomas—had little use of his arms or legs due to a stroke. He would kick and hit us because he wanted to go home and die, but his family forced him to come. He would allow me to place his needles as he sat weeping out of humiliation and longing for death.

Bob Domingo—had lost a leg to diabetes. He was dubbed a "slow code" by the techs. I was told he would be better off dead, so I shouldn't rush if he coded.

Eleanor and Evelyn—the two ladies who told me I would be an excellent teacher.

The Judge— one of the first African American judges in California. He went in for heart surgery and came out paralyzed from the chest down with kidney failure.

Dr. Richards—one of San Diego's most renowned physicians. The most afraid to die. He told me I had great hands every time I placed his needles. Terry—the white supremacist. Theresa—the mentally disabled woman who befriended me from the beginning cheering when she found out I was staying on at the unit after my training. One day she became very ill and spent an extended amount of time in the ICU. She came back with hospital-induced psychosis. She never spoke to me again. Just stared into space. The Iranian—The Russian—we almost killed that fucker with an air embolism. He never knew. The sixteen-year-old-- Dennis—Fay Carmello -- Mr. Mancini-- Mr. Lucchesi—he claimed to be part of a large mob family. He cried when Rosa coded. The Hamburgler—the real Hamburgler from the first McDonald's commercials. Flavia Ruiz—had lost both legs and both arms to diabetes and had developed MRSA. Her family would not sign the papers to remove her from dialysis. The Hell's Angels guy. The ex-prostitute. Steven—the blind guy who would sing Kiss songs at the top of his lungs. Arturo— Juanita Cassissi—sat tied to a chair by the tubes as her husband suffered a heart attack in the lobby. The schizophrenics—we had three in the time I was there. They all thought we were trying to kill them. Judy Andrade—an outgoing and talkative woman. She suffered a stroke while on dialysis and returned unable to communicate.

Those are just a handful of my ghosts. Each of them became nothing more than a note in the book at the nurse's station that announced his or her passing. When I was still working as a dialysis tech, I would dream every night of these people. Now, I only dream of them once in a while. They are the ones who inspired me to teach. They are the ones who remind me when I sleep that in the midst of life we are in death.

Heart Song

A journey of the hopeless heart—not of the wandering soul
I never expected to love you like I do
My Lord, he knew it from the start—I was not able to be whole
I had not yet seen the perfect shape he had created that was you

A journey up then crashing down—deep inside each hopeless beat
I didn't know He placed a love that grew
A bow to His glorious, mighty crown—a kiss to His innocent feet
My Lord, He knew it from the start—this love was something new

A journey to the ends of earth—my heart followed His shadowy face
I never expected you to love me like you do
I found myself deep inside—my heart—He called this place
Not yet seeing He created me to gather the scattered pieces of you

A journey to my Father's home—revealed His loving truth
His love was there for all—not just a chosen few
It was no longer needed for me to roam—this cold and broken earth
He held us both together as waves crashed and cold winds blew

A journey of the hopeless heart—brought me to a familiar place
I saw my home was here with you
To find my Lord had been there at the start—to meet me face to face
At the edge of heaven—in the rising sun--its rays a golden hue

Just Write Something!

There are holes in my thoughts—I can't remember them all. Stuck in the swirling drain of my mind. There is something about who I was and who I have become. There is something about my Baby DeAngelo and his deep, deep sadness. Thoughts of hopelessness creep into my heart. Have I really changed or has all remained the same? Trapped in a wordless, far off place. Thoughts. Memories. Images. A mother who has lost her children. Too little—too late. The weight of sadness tears through my body. It takes all my strength to keep going sometimes. It takes everything I have to speak the words of hope and love to a child who has lost everything.

DeAngelo told me of a dream in which he and I were trapped in a house as a scary man entered through the front door. In his dream he ran down the stairs to grab a gun—only to shoot himself—the bullet tearing through his head and coming to a stop halfway out of his forehead.

Half alive and half dead

I know how it feels to be half alive and half dead. I asked him why he shot himself instead of the scary man. DeAngelo replied, "So I wouldn't have to see him anymore." Sadly—I understood what he meant. I have encountered that man many times. He is always just around the corner—just behind the door—and just a dream away.

Dreaming

I do not dream in color, nor in black and white, but in the subtle tones of sepia's reddish golden light that casts a spell of madness across this mind of mine as it looks for clues and answers to life's quest for the sublime.

As day falls into watery night my thoughts fall carelessly close to a world that swallows up its prey—the ones it loves the most. For in my dreams I've lived a thousand lifetimes and died a thousand deaths. I've been lost on roads of loneliness and felt a thousand lover's breaths. There are some I don't remember, and some I'd just as soon forget, but it's the one's that keep returning that fill me with regret.

That house upon the ocean that I always seem to lose. The test with all wrong answers no matter what I choose. Roads that lead to nowhere and people I can't find. A break in my recovery causes my thoughts to hit rewind. So, I live them over and over, never remembering how they end. It's like a vicious circle carrying messages my mind forgets to send.

Freed for Adoption

The court dismissed the appeal on the decision to terminate the birth parents' parental rights today—freeing them for adoption. We will be able to adopt the boys by mid-May. They will be Isaiah Lee Baker Brazzi and DeAngelo Harris Brazzi. So awesome! I am so excited!

Thank you, Lord, for clearing a path I was unable to see. Please continue to guide and protect us as a family. Hold our hands as we cross this finish line into our new life as a family.

—Amen

It is the journey out of the darkness of isolation where we learn the most. Anyone can step into the forest, but finding the way back out often feels impossible—especially as night falls. I spent many nights there. Alone.

I do not have OCD! OCD has me!

Rachael-

Occasionally it allows me to walk freely among the other souls just so I can get a taste of how it feels to be real, but OCD never fails to pull me back into its protective arms, and it never fails to remind me that none of it is real. It is all a mirage--smoke and mirrors--a dream. It can all disappear in the blink of an eye, but more specifically, in the blink of my eye. The curtain is lifted away and I can see everything at once. Every possibility becomes a probability. You do not understand. There is no in between for me. I am either in the cold, dark forest of chaos, or I am in the parched, unforgiving desert of rigidity. I have been dragging myself along the burning landscape for too long this time and I cannot resist the water I see on the horizon. I must walk in that direction.

OCD makes it hard to get out of the shower because I cannot get the soap clean enough. Yes, that's right; the soap is not clean enough. Neither is the towel. Both wait patiently to contaminate the next person with my sexually transmitted diseases even though I have none. OCD makes it hard to get out of the bathroom because I cannot drink the right amount of water and I cannot set the glass in the right place in relation to my medication. If I drink only one sip, then I will be left with no one but myself. If I drink two sips, then I will be left with just myself and Jack. If I drink three sips, then I will be left with just myself, Jack and Grant. Five sips of water in just the right amounts. "That's right," whispers OCD, "just do it. You will feel better." OCD makes it hard to breathe because I need to take in a certain amount of air to create a certain feeling or else I might forget to breathe at all. I might not notice I have stopped breathing. OCD makes it hard to get out of the car because I have probably left someone or something in there that will suffocate in the heat. I can crack the windows. I can check to make sure I didn't really bring anyone but myself. I can check to make sure nothing snuck into my car while I wasn't looking, but I am never fully satisfied that I am not committing murder every single time I leave my car. OCD makes it hard to go to sleep because I have not worded my protective prayer correctly or I have not held my hands correctly or I have not been facing the right direction or I have forgotten someone. There is more, but that is all I can get out for now.

I hate having OCD! OCD makes it hard to love, hard to have hope, and hard to experience happiness. OCD makes it hard to be alive.

I am still recovering from the person I was for so long. I am still returning to the person I was in the beginning. Sometimes it is tempting to turn away from everything I have learned and everything I have gained.

I have often said I fear the ending of this story, but now that fear is gone. I know how this story ends. It ends with the sun rising on a new day—with a moment of absolute hope—a lion rising to devour the darkness of the night—preying on each and every lie the devil told me. I have found that, in this broken world, there is more heaven than hell—more beauty than ugly and the love is always greater than the hate. The despair of the night is always defeated by the hope of the rising sun as it beats back the demons of the cold, dark night. When all is said and done, I know I can say love finally won.

Thank you, Lord!

—Amen

<u>We finalized the adoption today! I am now the mother of three sons!</u>

Follow up to Pieces of Me

The Vibrant Leader—a mirror to your soul. She is intelligent, confident, and strikingly familiar. The person you have always wanted to meet, and in whom you see a part of yourself, stands before you looking you straight in the eye. She is knowledgeable, passionate, and daringly bold. The teacher you have always wanted to have who helps you forge a new path in your head...and your heart holds your hand as you prepare to move forward. She is articulate, eloquent and movingly spoken. The speaker you have always wanted to see who says the things you have always longed to hear is taking the stage.

I am still a leader, not because I have to take control, but because I am better at stepping back. I am still a mirror, but now I can see my own reflection in others. They are windows to my soul and they teach me more than I could have ever imagined and lead me to places I didn't know existed.

The Faithful Worshipper—a carrier of hope. She is white-hot and on fire with the Holy Spirit. The Christian you have always hoped really exists walks into your life. She is brave and courageous—a risk taking soldier for the Lord. The warrior you want fighting on your side, who would lay down this temporary life in order to save your eternal one, shields you with the Lord's greatest weapon: LOVE. She is a compassionate, never-tiring servant. The missionary you pray knocks on the door of your mud hut...in your town without water or food or electricity to bring a spark of hope to your darkness has arrived.

I am still a carrier of hope, but because of my darkness, not because of my light. My story allows me to bring God's hope and love into a world that is falling apart. I am still a faithful worshipper, not because I have blind faith, but because I have experienced losing it. I am still a warrior, not because I fought and lived, but because I surrendered and died. I must try to remember that I have surrendered and no longer need to fight. Sometimes I forget.

The Family Member—a wife, a mother, a daughter. She is devoted, understanding, and loving. The mother you wish were yours holds you and kisses you as she wipes away the tears. She is inadequate, unpredictable, and shockingly explosive. The mother you wish were dead crushes you with words. She is committed and faithful. The wife you want as your partner in life lies by your side and caresses your soul as you dream. She is hateful and unforgiving. The wife you should leave, but are afraid to let go of, begins to walk out the door yet never makes it out of the hallway. She is perfect and successful. A fake daughter you will never really know who stands like a porcelain doll on your shelf—beautiful yet so easily broken.

I am still a loving mother, but one who wipes away the tears of skinned knees, not the tears of crushing shame. I am enough when I love with my whole heart. Actually, I am a totally kick ass mom. I am now the mother I wish I had.

I am still a committed and faithful wife, but I have learned the freedom of forgiveness and the healing power of love. We left that hallway and walked out that door together. We have a beautiful life together—even though I have a highly intense husband. Apparently I like intensity.

I am still a perfect and successful daughter, but at least I have told my parents how I have been broken by life and glued back together by the small hands of my children. It is not my fault if they are too blind to see the cracks.

The Friend—a confidante and comrade. She is funny and uplifting and causes you to understand what C.S. Lewis meant when he said, "The typical expression of opening friendship would be something like, 'What? You too? I thought I was the only one." Someone who can always make you smile as you walk together down a secret path known only to the two of you. She is deeply connected yet always keeps you at an arm's length. You discover that the friend you've been searching for is trapped behind a plate of glass as you reach in for a hug. Don't get too close to her heart. You might make it skip a beat...you might make it care.

Even in my fear, I have always been a good friend. I have always cared. The closeness of friendship no longer burns—no longer suffocates. I have started to let people into my life, and I have found that people are more accepting than I thought.

The Shadow—a glimmer of a human being. She is frozen, afraid, and desperately alone. Unable to speak, the suicide you never noticed, or could never force yourself to watch, weeps silently. She is weak, trembling, and hoping it will all go away. Like a shadow, flickering in and out of the rays of sunlight, cowering in the dimly lit hallway of an abandoned building, she is sad and hopeless in her ignorance and isolation. A stumbler, unable to find the light switch or the door, who finally escapes into the daybreak only to fall to the ground for the last time beaten and burned into nothingness by the violent, unforgiving sun as she realizes <u>she cannot survive being exposed</u>.

I will always remember the exact moment I thought my only option was death. At the time I could see no other options. I could not bear to live the next 40+ years half in and half out of this world. This part is a good reminder of where drugs take me. I am no longer a shadow. Being exposed has made me a living, breathing human being. I have the warmth of a loving family. I am never truly alone. I have every reason to live.

The Writer—a muse to your life. She is open and honest as the words flow freely from her fingers. There are no barriers to what she might say. Someone who will say the things the world needs to hear, but she just can't speak, is shouting through the megaphone of the page. She knows the Leader, the Worshipper, the Family Member, the Friend, and even the Shadow. She recognizes and accepts them all as essential parts of herself. The have helped her survive. They have helped her thrive. The writer is nothing without the brilliant light and even less without the smothering darkness. She is capable of being white-hot and stone-cold in the same moment because she knows the two are necessary to maintain balance and truth in her life.

I owe a lot to this part of myself. This one is probably what saved me because it forced me to be honest with myself. It was the one who said "help," the one who said "look," and the one who said, "now." The writer is the one who spoke when I couldn't. The writer is the one who pulled back the scab revealing the festering shame and exposing my best-kept secrets. The wound has begun to heal. I must remember to keep writing. Sometimes I forget.

The Loser—a stoner lost in time. She has her feet kicked up on the couch and can hang with anyone. The partier you have always wanted to laugh with, who knows how to work hard and play hard, sits on the floor as she rolls one up on your coffee table. She is cool and relaxed as she blazes through life, yet she, like the Writer, knows and accepts all the others. She knows them because she is *all of them all the time.* She feels and moves to the rhythm of life, and recognizing the oneness of the world and the eternal moment that is now. She is careless and couldn't care less. It is all good as she dissolves into creation and her edges soften.

I am no longer lost in time. I no longer want to be lost in time. I want to be there for every last second of every single day. I still have my feet kicked up on the couch, but I have learned to work less and play harder. I am not always cool and relaxed, and I am not blazing through life, but at least I am not going up in flames.

Dreams

In my dreams I am the person I used to be. I smoke, I drink, I travel. I see old friends and travel old streets, but they are never quite the same. I stay up all night. Insomnia and panic keep coming. I travel on flights across worlds and times only to realize I have not slept for days. I try to sleep, but I never do.

In my dreams it is always night. Sometimes it is just on the verge of daybreak. I am never safe, but I am always familiar with where I am. I have always been there before, but now I don't belong and now I can't remember which direction to go or how long I should stay.

In my dreams I am always searching. Always lost in places I should know. People and things are not where they should be. I find myself alone and searching. Sometimes I find my way. Sometimes someone shows me the way. Sometimes I remember where I am. Who I am.

I have been here before, but this is not where I should be.

In my dreams I am late for a birthday party. I am lost in a parking lot. I am shopping for something and unable to find it. I drive in cars with my children's birthmother. We work the maze of streets together looking for our children.

In my dreams I see dead tiny peacocks. I cannot find a baseball game, I am late or I forgot to study or I forgot to show up for a class. I am always in a place I have been before, but never in the right place at the right time.

In my dreams my teeth crumble. I know secret passageways through homes I do not belong in. It is always night. Sometimes the sun is just beginning to set. I search for people I never find. The freeways of San Diego are made of rushing water, and I have favorite roads to take.

I know where I am, but it is not where I am supposed to be.

Shame

When I get stuck in shame, I don't allow God to carry me out of my low places. Psalm 139 is a reminder that I cannot hide from Him.

Psalm 139

*1 O Lord, you have examined my heart
    and know everything about me.
2 You know when I sit down or stand up.
    You know my thoughts even when I'm far away.
3 You see me when I travel
    and when I rest at home.
    You know everything I do.
4 You know what I am going to say
    even before I say it, Lord.
5 You go before me and follow me.
    You place your hand of blessing on my head.
6 Such knowledge is too wonderful for me,
    too great for me to understand!
7 I can never escape from your Spirit!
    I can never get away from your presence!
8 If I go up to heaven, you are there;
    if I go down to the grave, you are there.
9 If I ride the wings of the morning,
    if I dwell by the farthest oceans,
10 even there your hand will guide me,
    and your strength will support me.
11 I could ask the darkness to hide me
    and the light around me to become night—
12   but even in darkness I cannot hide from you.
To you the night shines as bright as day.
    Darkness and light are the same to you.
13 You made all the delicate, inner parts of my body
    and knit me together in my mother's womb.
14 Thank you for making me so wonderfully complex!*

Your workmanship is marvelous—how well I know it.
15 You watched me as I was being formed in utter seclusion,
   as I was woven together in the dark of the womb.
16 You saw me before I was born.
   Every day of my life was recorded in your book.
Every moment was laid out
   before a single day had passed.
17 How precious are your thoughts about me, O God.
   They cannot be numbered!
18 I can't even count them;
   they outnumber the grains of sand!
And when I wake up,
   you are still with me!
23 Search me, O God, and know my heart;
   test me and know my anxious thoughts.
24 Point out anything in me that offends you,
   and lead me along the path of everlasting life.

Why don't I allow God to do His work through me?

Because:

God asks me to do hard things
He asks me to go where no one else wants to go
Sometimes I get tired, so I close my eyes and my ears to His calling
Sometimes I stop caring
Sometimes I lose faith
Sometimes it feels like He is not there
Satan shouts, but God whispers. Sometimes it is hard to hear Him
through all the noise

However:

God also gives me everything I need to accomplish those hard things
And He also walks with me into those hard places
And He holds me when I sleep
And He cares until I can again

And He knows difficult things will cause my faith to grow
And He is always there. I just need to look closer

So, I must find some time each day when I can sit and listen to Him

Restless Sky

The restless sky it welcomes me
I see it deep behind my eye—trails of reds and blues
With arms outstretched it begs for me to leap from its horizons
Where angels learn to fly and devils pay their dues

The crushing tide it beckons me
I feel waves thrashing in my mind—pounding of water on sand
With arms outstretched it begs for me to swim from its shores
Where beauty goes to die and fate reaches out its hand

The silent earth it calls for me
I hear it echoing in my heart—cries of future and past
With arms outstretched it begs for me to climb its mountain tops
Where life departs and each breath becomes my last

The burning flame it welcomes me
I smell it tearing through my soul—embers of old and new
With arms outstretched it begs for me to dance in its light
Where evil turns to coal and I rise from ash anew

Amaya

The Lord has spoken again! We got guardianship of Amaya, the boys' cousin, one day after her tenth birthday. She is going to St. Joseph's and has made some great friends. She has escaped a lifetime of homelessness and abuse. It is time for her to begin healing. I know the Lord has some amazing plans for this fierce little girl.

A girl! Wow! I never thought I would ever actually have the daughter I had envisioned over the years. She is amazing, resilient, beautiful, funny, intelligent, curious, sassy, loving and connected. She is the final piece in this part of the puzzle—the final orange flower—revealing the family God had planned for me from the beginning. I saw them playing on the riverbank in the soft glow of the rising sun—and they were holding hands. Each has given me a special gift that only they could give.

The Life I would have Missed

I stand in utter amazement at the life I would have missed:

I would have missed DeAngelo's wavy black hair and his sly sense of humor. I would have missed Isaiah's sparkling smile and his charm and compassion. I would have missed Amaya's beauty and her brilliant plan to escape a life of hopelessness.

Grant, I would have known, but only as a little boy. I would have missed him as a man, a husband, a father. I would have missed hearing about his first kiss and his big dreams. I would not have seen this beautiful young man he is becoming.

I would have missed adoption. This home. This husband. This family. These friends. This life I would have missed.

I stop to take a look around at the life I would have missed
Had I stood a moment longer at the edge of the abyss
Had I listened one more second to the devil's hateful hiss
Had I closed my eyes forever—sealed by death's final kiss
Had I not heard the pounding of God's angry, mighty fists
Had I not turned around to see I had been made just for this

These Children

These children—they are not mine to keep
I drown in self-reliance and suffocate on self-sufficiency. I destroyed
myself by thinking I was enough to save them from the deepest seas
and the towering waves.

These children—they are not mine to have
I turn their faces in God's direction—so—when they return home to
Him—He will say, "I know you," and they will respond, "We know
you, too!"

These children—they are not mine to save
My sin is not their sin. My darkness is not what they see. I destroyed
myself by thinking theirs was my path to pave along the way.

These children—they are mine to love
I turn their gazes to the sun and wrap my arms in hugs to hum a
sweet, sweet song of forevermore—so, when they see Him—they
will recognize the Lord.

As a child I always thought my fears would go away when I became an adult. I didn't know that grownups are afraid of the dark, too. It is only recently that I have come to be at peace with the demons which have haunted me. It is not that they have left. They remain, but today I no longer fear their power. They have brought me closer to the God they once told me had abandoned me. They have made me appreciate the children they once told me I didn't deserve. They have helped me to understand the child I once was.

Waking up from a lifelong death…a lifelong doom…is a little like waking up in heaven. The light carries with it a subtle shimmer. A glorious glow buzzing through the atmosphere. The quiet carries with it a gentle peace that flows deeper than any wave of sound ever heard. There is a flicker of joy so intense it blinds me to the broken pieces of the world. There is a hope that holds it all together…and I can see it clearly now.

The Lord expects nothing of me, but He has given me great things to do in His name. He sat with me in the darkest shadows of my heart and He smiled because He knew the plans He had for me. He saw only the beauty that was to come.

When death gasps its final breath, I will be there to watch it go. The promise of tomorrow will not be needed because all hope—all joy— will be grasped tightly in the grip of today. The sunrise I have traveled so far to see will break above the mountain and I will be blinded by its beauty as I watch God's children play at heaven's edge.

Heaven and hell do not intersect. They collide. Heaven and hell do not coexist. One crushes the other. I stand at the point where life tramples death. I do not have to choose between the two because I do not have a choice. In the end love wins and we discover we are all headed home no matter where we stand.

1 Corinthians 13:1-8

If I speak in the tongues of men or of angels, but do not have love, I am only a resounding gong or a clanging cymbal.

If I have the gift of prophecy and can fathom all mysteries and all knowledge, and if I have a faith that can move mountains, but do not have love, I am nothing.

If I give all I possess to the poor and give over my body to hardship that I may boast but do not have love, I gain nothing.

Love is patient, love is kind. It does not envy, it does not boast, it is not proud. It does not dishonor others, it is not self-seeking, it is not easily angered. It keeps no record of wrongs. Love does not delight in evil but rejoices with the truth.

It always protects, always trusts, always hopes, always perseveres.

<u>Love never fails</u>

Acknowledgement

"Suicide is Painless" Composer Johnny Mandell. Used by permission of Alfred Publishing. All rights reserved. Any third-party use, outside of this publication, is prohibited.